实用急救教程

Practical First Aid Manual

主　编　韩　伟　李景波　陈向东

科学出版社

北　京

内 容 简 介

本书共10章，围绕应急救护、急救相关法律知识、心肺复苏及AED的使用、创伤现场救护、常见意外伤害救护、常见急症救护、灾难逃生与救护、心理急救、妊娠期健康及感染控制与预防措施相关内容展开，旨在帮助读者在面对各种意外伤害事件和突发急症场景下快速做出反应，实施科学而有效的急救措施，避免因急救人员失误导致更严重的情况发生。

本书内容通俗易懂，图片丰富生动，可供对急救相关知识感兴趣的在校学生及公众学习参考。

图书在版编目（CIP）数据

实用急救教程 / 韩伟，李景波，陈向东主编. —北京：科学出版社，2023.7

ISBN 978-7-03-074420-3

Ⅰ.①实… Ⅱ.①韩…②李…③陈… Ⅲ.①急救–教材 Ⅳ.①R459.7

中国版本图书馆CIP数据核字（2022）第251371号

责任编辑：马晓伟 路 倩 / 责任校对：张小霞
责任印制：赵 博 / 封面设计：吴朝洪

科学出版社 出版
北京东黄城根北街16号
邮政编码：100717
http://www.sciencep.com

涿州市殷润文化传播有限公司印刷
科学出版社发行 各地新华书店经销
*
2023年7月第 一 版 开本：787×1092 1/16
2024年8月第二次印刷 印张：13
字数：170 000
定价：68.00元
（如有印装质量问题，我社负责调换）

《实用急救教程》
编写人员

主 编　韩　伟　李景波　陈向东
副主编　杨　乐
编 者　（按姓氏汉语拼音排序）

陈向东	范　斌	冯　媛	韩　溟
韩　伟	何　慧	黄敏强	姬忠良
冷少龙	李　丹	李　朋	李景波
林萍萍	刘　伟	刘小凤	彭　净
丘坚成	阮中瑞	陶　倩	王　鑫
王双卫	王焱芬	温　强	吴　强
杨　乐	杨玉娇	曾佳凡	张卫文
赵聚钊	郑　莉	钟海燕	

序 言

突发事件包括自然灾害、事故灾难、公共卫生事件等，具有突然性、不确定性、社会性等特点，是世界各国不得不面临的现实课题之一。21世纪以来，全球突发事件呈多发、频发态势，如地震、飓风、火灾、爆炸、恐怖活动和传染性疾病的流行，尤其是2019年末暴发的新型冠状病毒感染疫情，成为第二次世界大战以来对世界影响重大的灾难事件之一。

我国是世界上自然灾害最为严重的国家之一，灾害种类多，分布地域广，发生频率高，造成损失重，这是一个基本国情。目前世界正处于大发展、大变革和大调整时期，加强各类突发事件的管理和应对，对全面建成社会主义现代化强国，全面推进中华民族伟大复兴具有极其重要的意义。

目前，我国大部分公民普遍缺乏灾难或意外伤害等急救知识，在紧急情况下往往不知所措或操作不当，导致伤病情不同程度延误。据有关数据显示，我国公民在急救知识普及、对急救技能的掌握方面整体还落后于发达国家。研究证实，当遭遇严重意外创伤或危及生命的突发疾病时，伤病员的存活率及预后与现场救治是否及时、恰当有直接关系，学习急救相关知识有可能挽救身边的生命和减少伤残，因此向公众普及急救知识，提高群众自救互救能力成为当务之急。

2018年10月，深圳大学总医院急诊科牵头成立了公众急救培训小组，定期向学校、社区等单位组织"全民救心"公益急救培训活动，引起广大市民的热烈反响和高度称赞。为进一步普及应急救护知识，提升公众应急救护技能，深圳大学总医院急救团队本着"人人学急救，急救为人人"的理念，总结和提炼了团队多年的工作经验，对标国际急救标准编写了《实用急救教程》一书。该书力求呈现最新、规范、有效的急救知识，为急救培训提供参考。全书共十章，内容涵盖心肺复苏、创伤、溺水、触电等常见急诊伤病的紧急处置方法，实用、易学。希望该书能够在推广急救知识、加强公众应急救护意识和对急救技能的掌握上发挥积极作用。

　　面对处于危难中的生命，鼓励公众敢放手、施援手，是社会进步的应有之义。而让公众"有一手"、会援手，将掌握医疗急救常识作为必备技能，也应该是现代社会中公民的能力标配。希望该书能帮助解决公众遇到突发意外伤害时不敢救、不会救、救不了的问题；使现场应急救护体系更加普及化、系统化，真正让施救者"敢救、会救、能救"，并让更多公众参与到应急救护技能的传播中；以点带面，带动整个社会增强公众应急救护意识，提高公众自救互救能力和防灾避险技能。

　　该书内容丰富、通俗易懂，具有很高的实践指导价值，可帮助读者积累急救知识，面对危险能快速反应，为生命救治争取宝贵时间。

侯世科

天津大学应急医学研究院院长

中华医学会灾难医学分会主任委员

2022年6月

目录 / Contents

第一章

应急救护概述

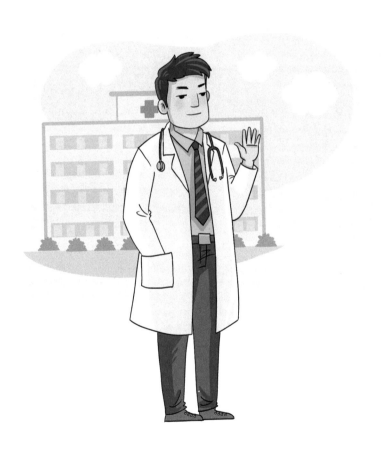

一、定　义

急救，即应急救护，指在突发伤病或灾害事故的现场，在专业人员到达之前，为伤病员提供初步、及时、有效的救护措施。

二、特　点

急救是现场的、初级的、群众性的应急救护。

三、目　的

1. 挽救生命

采取任何急救措施挽救伤病员的生命。

2. 防止恶化

防止伤情继续发展和二次伤害，减轻伤残。

3. 促进恢复

促进伤病员身体和心理的康复。

四、救护原则

1. 保证安全

排除危险因素，确保环境安全；做好自我防护，戴医用防护手套，必要时穿防护服。

2. 防止感染

避免直接接触伤病员的分泌物、血液、体液等。

3. 合理救护

先救命后治伤；迅速判定有无头、胸、腹部致命伤；保持气道通畅；先止血后包扎。

五、正 确 呼 救

争分夺秒开展应急救护的同时，应尽快拨打"120"急救电话，也可以向周围群众呼救寻求帮助。

电话报告内容：

（1）伤病员所在的具体地点、周边明显的标志物和建筑等。

（2）伤病员的年龄、性别、人数等。

（3）伤病员的基本情况，如大出血、昏迷不醒、胸痛、呕吐、呼吸困难等。

（4）发生意外的可能原因，如交通事故、溺水、触电、中毒等。

（5）报告人的姓名和电话号码。

（6）问清救护车到达的大致时间，做好接车准备。

一定要清楚准确地回答电话接听者的问话，并等接听者告知可以结束时，再挂断电话。

第二章

急救相关法律知识

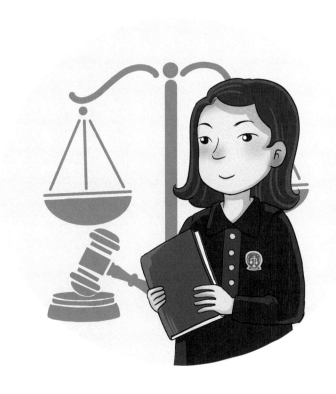

本章介绍的急救相关法律保障和风险，均仅指社会急救，即由非医疗急救人员现场实施的救护患者的活动。

见义勇为、危难之时伸手帮扶，历来是中华民族的优良传统。遗憾的是，多年以来，让英雄流血又流泪的事件屡屡发生，甚至助人者惹上法律纠纷，使普通民众对施救产生顾虑。

2017年10月1日起《中华人民共和国民法总则》正式实施，其中被俗称为"好人法"的第一百八十四条规定：因自愿实施紧急救助行为造成受助人损害的，救助人不承担民事责任（《民法总则》废止后，该条文在《中华人民共和国民法典》第一百八十四条中体现）。自2018年10月1日起施行的《深圳经济特区医疗急救条例》第五十一条规定：在医疗急救人员到达前，鼓励现场具备急救能力的人员实施紧急救护。由此可见，政府对此是持明确鼓励态度的。

当然，仅仅鼓励是不够的。普通民众在不负有法律义务的情况下，作为施救者来施救，还至少面临以下问题。

第一，如果我施救了，但被救者未被救活，或者在施救过程中对被救者造成了二次伤害，该怎么办？

2013年8月1日起施行的《深圳经济特区救助人权益保护规定》第四条规定：被救助人主张救助人在救助过程中未尽合理限度注意义务加重其人身损害的，应当提供证据予以证明。没有证据证明或者证据不足以证明其主张的，依法由被救助人承担不利后果。从中可以看出，如果施救者在施救的过程中已经尽到了自己的合理限度注意义务，即便是造成了损害，也是不承担法律责任的。

第二，如果我施救却反被诬陷，该怎么办？

《深圳经济特区救助人权益保护规定》第三条规定：被救助人主张其人身损害是由救助人造成的，应当提供证据予以证明。没有证据或者证据不足以证明其主张的，依法由被救助人承担不利后果。第五条规定：救助人因被救助人捏造事实，诬告陷害而发生费用的，有权依法向被救助人追偿。第六条规定：被救助人捏造事实，诬告陷害救助人，构成违反治安管理规定行为的，依法予以行政处罚；构成犯罪的，依法追究刑事责任。被救助人捏造事实，诬告陷害救助人的，救助人可以向人民法院提起民事诉讼，要求被救助人承担赔礼道歉、赔偿损失、消除影响、恢复名誉等民事责任。

第三，如果我施救了，我本人在施救过程中受到了伤害怎么办？

自2013年1月1日起施行的《广东省见义勇为人员奖励和保障条例》，对于被认定为见义勇为的人员给予了全面的保护，既有精神、荣誉方面的，也包括比较全面的经济保障，如医疗费等。

综上所述，为免除施救者的后顾之忧，规定对患者实施的善意的、无偿的、合乎常理的紧急救护行为受法律保护，其责任予以免除。

但需要强调的是，无论何时何地，作为不负有法律救助义务的普通公民，需要牢记的重要原则：在确保自身安全的前提下施救。如果经评估后有风险，或者自己没有能力完成救助行为的，建议及时拨打"110"报警或者拨打"120"通知专业急救人员。

第三章

心肺复苏及AED的使用

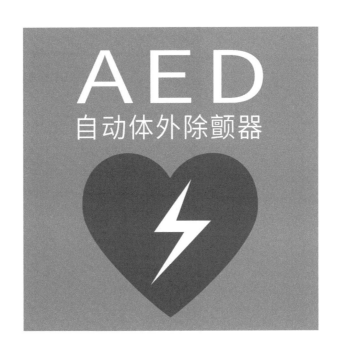

心搏骤停已成为当前相当严重的公共健康问题，是世界上许多地区的主要死亡原因之一。心搏骤停在医院内外均可发生。本章重点介绍非医务人员在医院外进行心肺复苏（CPR）所需要掌握的基本知识和技能，以期提高危急状态下生命的抢救成功率。基础生命支持程序为C—A—B（胸外按压—开放气道—人工呼吸）。

第一节　成人心肺复苏

成人心肺复苏步骤

1. 评估

（1）确保现场对急救人员和患者都是安全的。

（2）轻拍患者的肩膀，并大声呼唤："你还好吗？"

（3）评估患者是否有反应。

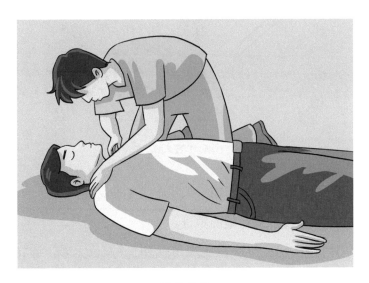

评估患者

2. 启动应急反应系统并获得自动体外除颤器（AED）

（1）寻求他人帮助，拨打急救电话。

（2）派人去拿或获得AED。

3. 评估呼吸

用5～10秒观察胸廓起伏情况，如果没有起伏则评估为心搏骤停。

4. 开始周期CPR

施救者应当采用"30次按压∶2次人工通气"的按压－通气比例。

胸部按压技术：

（1）施救者跪或站到患者一侧，双腿分开。

（2）确保患者仰卧在坚固的平坦表面上，确保患者头部、颈部和躯干保持在一条直线上。

（3）将一只手的掌根放在患者胸部正中央。

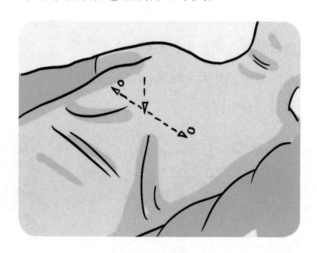

胸部按压位置

（4）将另一只手的掌根置于第一只手上，并交叉紧握。

（5）伸直双臂，使双臂与地面垂直。

（6）用力快速按压，每次按压深度达到5～6cm，每分钟100～120次，确保胸壁完全回弹，尽量减少中断。

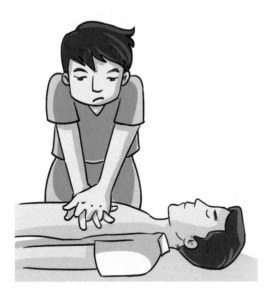

胸部按压姿势

（7）开放气道进行人工通气。首先清理气道，然后开放气道。开放气道采用仰头提颏法或推举下颌法。可采用口对口人工呼吸或口对面罩通气法（也可使用球囊面罩），每次人工通气应该使胸部隆起，确认为有效通气。

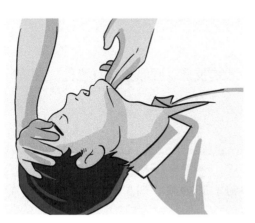

仰头提颏法

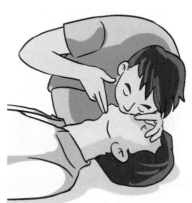

口对口人工呼吸

第二节 儿童、婴儿心肺复苏

一、儿童心肺复苏步骤

1. 评估现场环境

2. 启动应急反应系统并获得 AED

3. 检查患儿呼吸和反应

用 5～10 秒观察患儿胸腹部，如果没有明确感受到起伏（即没有呼吸），则从胸外按压开始 CPR（C—A—B 程序）。

4. 开始周期 CPR

单人施救者应采用"30 次按压：2 次人工通气"的按压-通气比例。双人则采用 15：2 的按压-人工通气比例。每次按压深度约 5cm，频率 100～120 次 / 分，确保胸壁完全回弹，尽量减少中断。最后开放气道，再进行两次人工通气。

二、婴儿心肺复苏步骤

1. 评估现场环境

检查婴儿是否有反应和呼吸，如果没有反应、呼吸或仅有喘息，应呼叫帮助。

2. 启动应急反应系统并获得 AED

3. 检查婴儿呼吸

用 5～10 秒观察胸腹部起伏，如果没有明确感受到起伏（即没有呼吸），则从胸外按压开始 CPR（C—A—B 程序）。

4. 心肺复苏

（1）单手胸外心脏按压：用双指按压，将两根手指放在婴儿胸部中央，乳头连线正下方，不要按压胸骨下端，应当采用"30 次按压：2 次人工通气"

的按压－通气比例。

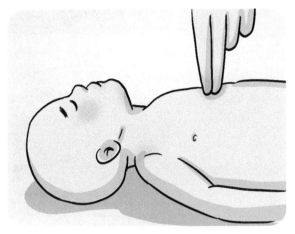

单手胸外心脏按压

（2）双拇指环绕法：将两个拇指并排放在婴儿胸部中央的胸骨下半部，双手环绕婴儿胸部，并以其余手指支撑婴儿的背部。采用15：2的按压－通气比例。

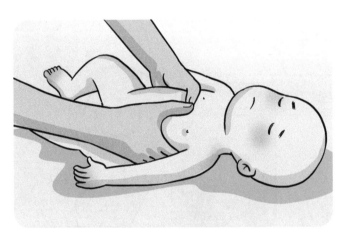

双拇指环绕法

每次按压深度大约4cm（胸壁前后径的1/3），频率100～120次/分，确保胸壁完全回弹，尽量减少中断。

5. 开放气道进行人工通气

采用仰头提颏法开放气道，并给予口对口呼吸或口对面罩通气。

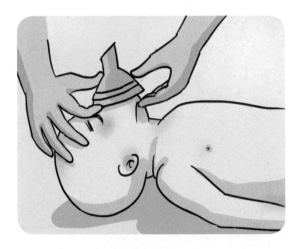

口对面罩通气

第三节　AED 的使用

AED操作流程：

（1）打开AED。

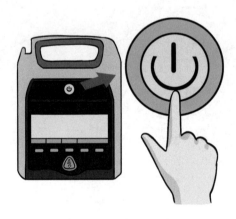

打开电源

（2）将与患者年龄相符的合适尺寸的电极片按图示贴在正确位置，并连接导联线。

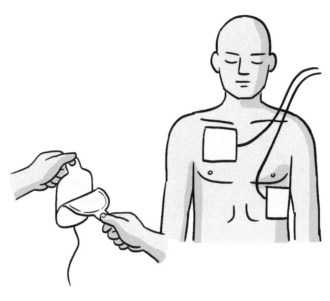

贴电极片

（3）遣散患者周围的人员，使用AED分析心律。

（4）根据AED提示，如需电击，则按下"充电"按钮，充电结束确认所有人离开后，按下"放电"按钮，而后立即进行CPR，如提示"无需电击"，则继续进行CPR。

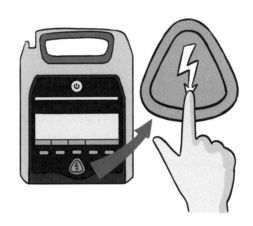

电击

（5）CPR过程中不要关闭AED。

（6）在施以电击时确保施救者处于安全环境。

（7）如为双人心肺复苏，在AED分析阶段，施救者应交换角色。

第四章

创伤现场救护

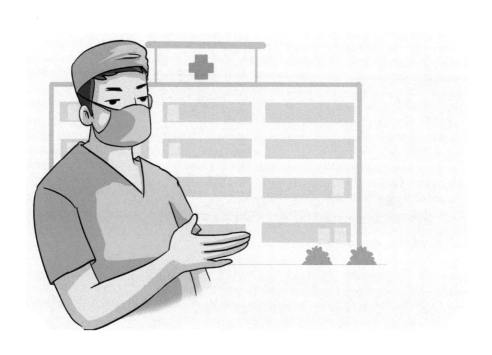

　　创伤主要是指机械力作用于人体所造成的损伤。创伤是一个既古老又年轻的医学课题。说它古老，是因为自人类诞生之日起，就开始出现创伤；说它年轻，是因为随着社会进步和医学发展，创伤却有增无减，并被称为现代文明的"孪生兄弟"。

　　依照体表结构的完整性是否受到破坏，可将创伤分为开放性创伤和闭合性创伤两大类。现场对开放性创伤的正确处理可以减轻受伤者的伤害程度。下面这些急救手段可有效地帮助大家正确处理开放性创伤。

第一节　开放性创伤后出血的处理

　　开放性创伤包括皮肤破损、血管及神经断裂、骨折等，出血非常常见，其中肉眼可见的为外出血，只要不是大动脉出血，受伤者得救的机会往往比较大。创伤止血最常用的方法是加压包扎止血法，头部、四肢及身体各处的伤口都可使用该方法。在无法立即就医的情况下，该方法可以马上派上用场。

一、正确的止血方法

1. 直接压迫伤口

　　用一块足够厚、足够大、清洁的敷料，持续不断地压住伤口，敷料范围应超出伤口3～4cm。

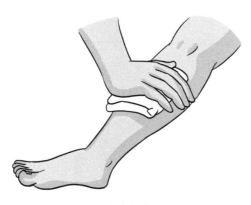

压迫止血

2. 指压止血法

用手指压在出血动脉近心端（离心脏近的地方）附近的骨头上，阻断血流来源，以达到止血目的。

（1）头顶部、颞部出血：在伤侧耳前，用示指或拇指压迫同侧耳前方颞浅动脉搏动点。

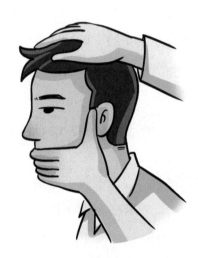

指压颞浅动脉

（2）面部出血：一侧颜面部出血，用示指或拇指压迫同侧面动脉搏动处。面动脉在下颌骨下缘下颌角前方约3cm处。

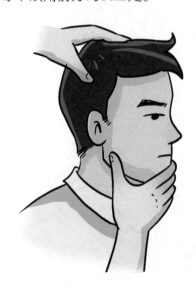

指压面动脉

（3）上肢出血：压迫腋动脉（腋窝部）或对着肱骨压迫肱动脉，并将患肢抬高。

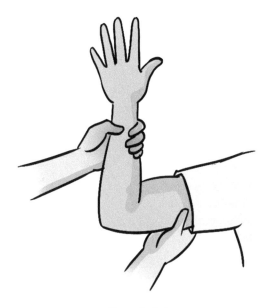

指压肱动脉

（4）手掌出血：在腕部压迫桡动脉、尺动脉。

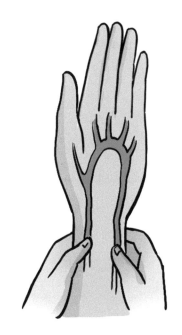

指压桡动脉、尺动脉

（5）手指出血：用拇指、示指同时压迫手指两侧动脉。

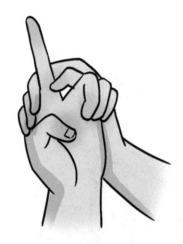

压迫指动脉

二、包　扎

应利用一切可以利用的消毒或清洁的软性材料，如毛巾、软布、衣物等，以达到及时包扎的目的。包扎的原则是先盖后包，力度适中。先盖后包，即先在伤口上盖上敷料（如够大、够厚的棉织品衬垫）或纱布，然后用绷带或三角巾包扎。力度适中即包扎后应止血有效，检查远端的动脉还在搏动；包扎过松，则止血无效；包扎过紧，则会造成远端组织缺血缺氧或坏死。

（一）加压包扎法

体表及四肢伤出血，大多数可通过加压包扎和抬高肢体达到暂时止血的目的。将无菌敷料或衬垫覆盖在伤口上，用手或其他物体在包扎伤口的敷料上施以压力，最常见的有加垫屈肘止血和加垫屈膝止血，一般需要持续5～15分钟才可奏效。同时，将受伤部位抬高也有利于止血，此法适用于小动脉，中、小静脉或毛细血管出血。

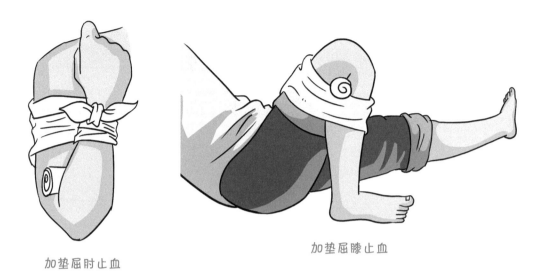

加垫屈肘止血　　　　加垫屈膝止血

如遇伤口内有异物，处理原则：①表浅异物可取；②深部异物不拔除（不取），固定异物并包扎。

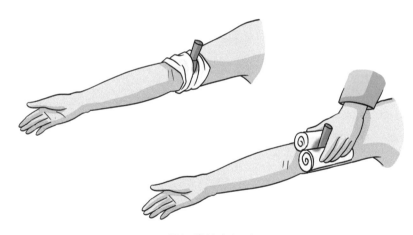

深部异物包扎法

如果遇到肢体伤口喷血，就要用止血带止血，可用布带、绳索、三角巾或毛巾替代，称为止血带止血法。也可加用一小棍插在活结内绞紧，称为布带绞紧止血法。

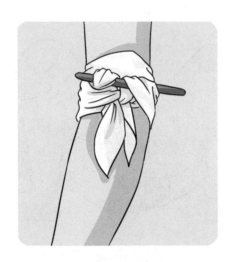

布带绞紧止血

此外，还可以使用腰带扣紧止血。

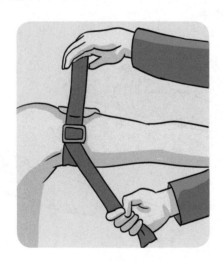

腰带扣紧止血

注意要点：带子下面要有衬垫，绞紧止血后记录时间，40分钟放松1次。塑料绳、电线、铁丝不可用。

（二）绷带包扎法

1. 环形包扎法

该方法适用于粗细相等的肢体及胸腹等处的包扎。

　　具体方法：将绷带作环形重叠缠绕，第一圈环绕稍作斜状，第二圈、第三圈作环形，并将第一圈斜出的一角压于环形圈内，这样固定更牢靠些。最后用胶布将尾部固定，或将带尾剪成两头打结。

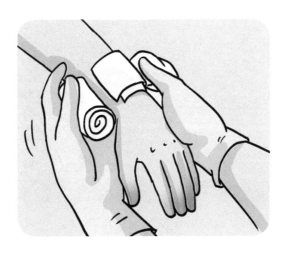

环形包扎法

2. 螺旋包扎法

该方法适用于粗细不相等的肢体的包扎。

　　具体方法：先按环形包扎法缠绕几圈固定，然后上缠，每圈盖住前圈的1/3或2/3，呈螺旋形。完全覆盖伤口后，原位缠绕两圈后固定。

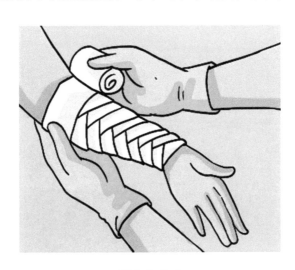

螺旋包扎法

3. "8"字包扎法

即在关节弯曲处上下两方，一圈向上、一圈向下呈"8"字形来回缠绕，每圈在弯曲处与前圈相交，同时根据情况与前圈重叠或压盖2/3。

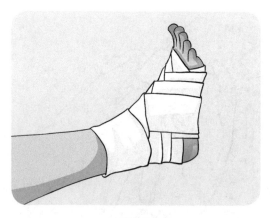

"8"字包扎法

4. 腹部开放伤口的包扎

如腹部有创伤伴脏器（如肠等）外露，包扎方法如下：①伤员取仰卧位，双腿屈曲，尽量使腹部肌肉松弛，以防内脏继续脱出；②对已脱出的内脏，先盖上干净塑料或敷料，四周用胶布固定，也可用一只干净的碗扣在其上，然后进行包扎；③严禁在急救时把脱出的内脏回纳至腹腔，以免造成腹腔感染。

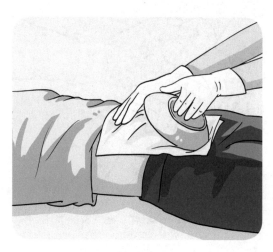

腹部创伤伴脏器外露包扎

注意要点：①在伤口处用加压包扎止血。较小的割伤或划伤，用聚维酮碘（即碘伏）消毒后，再用创可贴包好。②不要向伤口内撒任何消炎粉及其他粉状物，不要轻易拔出伤口上的刺入物。

第二节　创伤后骨折的处理

一、四肢骨折

骨折发生后，固定是创伤救护的一项基本任务。正确良好的固定能迅速减轻患者的疼痛，减少出血。现场可利用一切可以利用的材料，如夹板、杂志、硬纸板、木板、扁担、木棍、树枝、竹竿、铁棒，甚至可以使用皮带和外套等物品固定骨折部位。如果没有上述固定材料，也可将骨折的肢体与伤员的躯干或健肢相固定，使躯干或健肢起到夹板的临时固定作用。常见的骨折处理包括前臂及手骨折的固定、上臂骨折的固定、大腿骨折的固定及小腿骨折的固定。

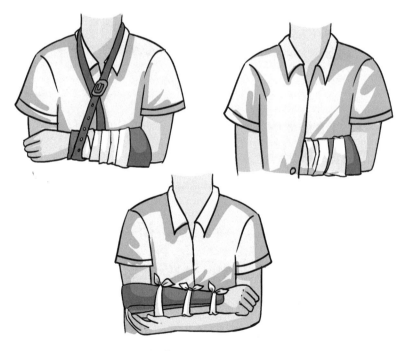

前臂及手骨折的固定

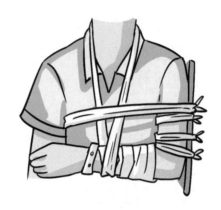

上臂骨折的固定

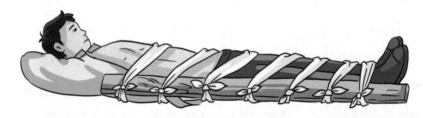

大腿骨折的固定

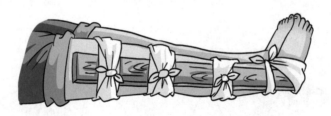

小腿骨折的固定

注意要点：①在肢体伤口处用加压包扎止血，并在现场寻找一切可用材料固定骨折的肢体，固定时注意要超过受伤肢体上下两个关节；②刺出皮肤的骨折端不要塞回皮肤内，原位包扎后固定。

二、脊柱骨折

创伤后脊柱局部疼痛、活动受限、畸形、压痛，甚至有不全或完全瘫痪的表现，如感觉和运动功能丧失、大小便功能障碍等，都要怀疑脊柱损伤，救治时要更加谨慎。在环境安全的前提下，切记不要轻易移动患者，时刻注意保持伤员的脊柱在一条轴线上。

可疑颈椎骨折的固定：可用两条毛巾卷置于颈部的两侧，然后绑在一起。注意松紧适当，不要影响呼吸。

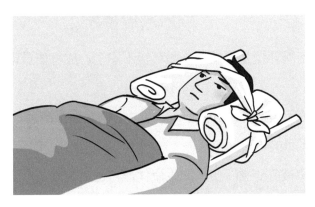

可疑颈椎骨折的固定

三、骨盆骨折

骨盆骨折是一种严重外伤，半数以上伴有并发症或多发伤，致残率极高，且如救治不当会有很高的死亡率。早期外固定对骨盆骨折引起的失血性休克的抢救十分有意义。

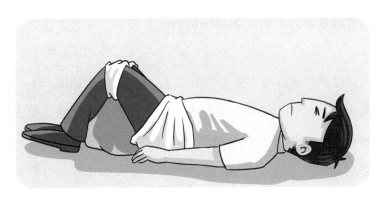

骨盆骨折的固定

第三节 伤员搬运

一、伤员搬运原则

（1）首先判断环境是否安全，如环境不安全，应将伤员带离危险区（紧急搬运）。

（2）在环境无危险时，应先止血、包扎、固定后再搬运。

（3）不要无目的地移动伤员。

（4）移动伤员前要判断伤员的生命体征，迅速检查头、颈、胸、腹、背部、四肢，如疑似脊柱损伤，需固定脊柱在一条轴线上后再搬运。

（5）动作要轻巧、迅速，避免不必要的震动。

（6）运送伤员时要随时观察伤员的意识、呼吸、出血等情况。

（7）向伤员解释运送的方法和目的，取得伤员的配合。

二、搬运方法

根据紧急程度分为紧急搬运和非紧急搬运，若意外现场存在潜在危险或环境，不宜就地施行急救，要将伤员搬运至较安全舒适的地方，等待医疗救援。

徒手搬运法是在搬运伤员的过程中仅凭人力而不使用器具的一种搬运方法。徒手搬运法包括单人搬运法、双人搬运法和多人搬运法。单人搬运法常包括衣服拖行法、被物拖行法、腋下拖行法等。对于怀疑脊柱损伤的伤员，不要轻易移动，应拨打急救电话，等待专业医疗人员（除非有充足的理由移动伤员）。

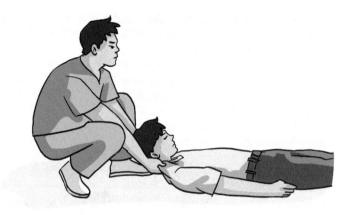

衣服拖行法

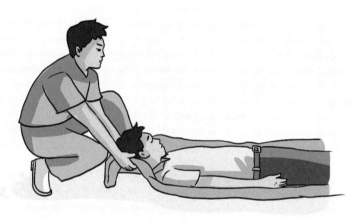

被物拖行法

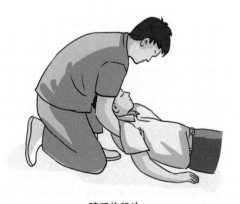

腋下拖行法

单人搬运法

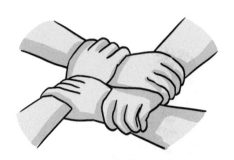

双人搬运法

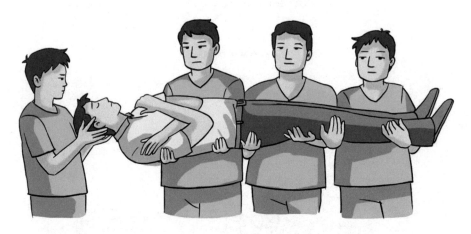

多人平托搬运法

第五章

常见意外伤害救护

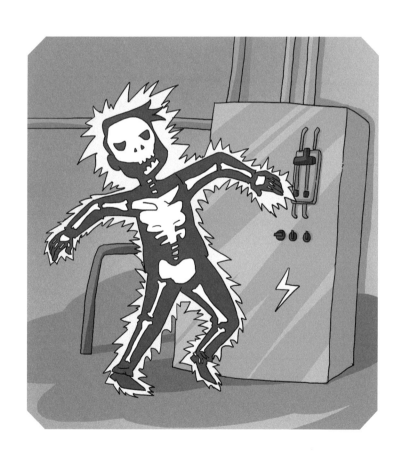

第一节 烧 烫 伤

一、概 述

烧烫伤指热力或间接热力（化学物质、电流、放射线等）作用于人体引起的组织损伤，主要指皮肤和黏膜损伤，严重者也可伤及皮肤和黏膜下组织结构，如肌肉、骨、关节甚至内脏。

二、表 现

烧伤深度可按三度四分法分为Ⅰ度、浅Ⅱ度、深Ⅱ度和Ⅲ度。

Ⅰ度烧伤：主要损害皮肤角质层，有局部轻度红肿，无水疱，疼痛明显。

浅Ⅱ度烧伤：可达真皮层，有水疱，疼痛剧烈。

深Ⅱ度烧伤：水疱小，但密度高，皮肤溃烂。

Ⅲ度烧伤：皮肤干燥，局部蜡白、焦黄或炭黑，疼痛消失。

小面积表浅烧伤，除了烧伤局部有红、肿、热、痛外，全身可以没有变化，如不感染，一般数天内痊愈。大面积深度烧伤，可以破坏人体内环境的稳定，出现全身各个系统的功能紊乱，如休克、肝肾功能异常，局部与全身感染、败血症，多器官功能不全、衰竭，乃至死亡。

三、救护措施

烧伤救护措施可总结为"1冲2脱3泡4盖5送"，不要涂抹药物。

第一步：冲

用冷水冲洗，或将烫伤的四肢浸泡在干净的冷水中，如此冲洗或浸泡15～30分钟，直至感受不到疼痛和灼热。

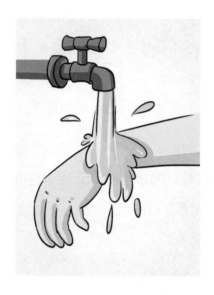

冲

第二步：脱

烫伤时若穿着贴身的衣物，要在冷水冲洗后脱除或使用剪刀剪开，小心除去衣物。不可强行剥去衣物，以免弄破水疱。摘掉烫伤部位附近的首饰。

第三步：泡

对于疼痛明显者，可将烫伤的肢体持续浸泡在冷水中10～30分钟，主要目的是缓解疼痛。

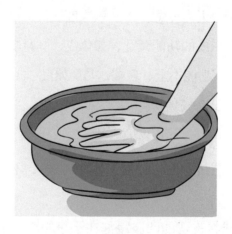

泡

第四步：盖

使用干净、无菌的纱布或棉质布类覆盖在伤口上，并加以固定，如此有助于保持创口清洁，减少外界的污染。

第五步：送

尽快将伤者送往医院进一步救治。

第二节　溺　　水

一、概　　述

（1）溺水是意外损伤导致死亡的常见原因，尤其是青少年。

（2）溺水导致死亡的主要原因是窒息缺氧。

（3）施救者应先确保自身安全，再尝试下水营救，盲目下水营救可能导致自身溺水。

（4）溺水急救应优先考虑开放气道和人工呼吸。

二、溺水生存链

（1）预防溺水：确保水中和周围安全。

（2）识别险情：呼喊他人寻求帮助。

（3）提供漂浮：避免下沉。

（4）脱离水域：只在安全时进行。

（5）提供必要护理：就医。

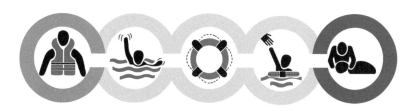

溺水生存链

三、未脱离水域营救措施

预防溺水	**确保水中和周围安全** （1）无论自己是在水中还是在水边上，需确保自己的手臂能够得着孩子 （2）在有救生员的安全水域游泳 （3）乘船只时穿救生衣 （4）学习游泳和水上安全生存技巧	
识别险情	**呼喊他人寻求帮助** （1）尽早识别溺水者的求救信号（溺水者可能并不会挥手或者呼救） （2）告诉别人打电话求助，自己留在现场提供援助	
提供漂浮	**避免下沉** **帮助他人时：** （1）远离水面以降低营救风险 （2）向溺水者扔漂浮物 **自救时：** （1）如果自己发生溺水，不要慌张，留在你可能拥有的任何漂浮物上 （2）如果可能的话，尽快发出求救信号，并漂浮起来	
脱离水域	**只在安全时进行** （1）帮助或指导溺水者自救，以脱离水域 （2）尽量在避免自己下水的情况下救出溺水者	
提供必要护理	**就医** （1）如果溺水者没有呼吸，应立即启动心肺复苏（通气和按压） （2）如果有条件，应考虑尽快使用供氧设备和AED （3）如果溺水者有呼吸，待在溺水者身边直到专业人员到来 （4）如出现任何症状，应寻求医疗援助，并对所有需要复苏的受害者进行急救	

四、脱离水域营救措施

确保安全	营救过程中先确保自身安全，切不可盲目下水
安抚溺水者	*安抚溺水者，鼓励和帮助他/她进行自我营救：* （1）不要心慌，一定要保持头脑清醒 （2）采取头顶向后，口向上方，将口鼻露出水面，此时能进行呼吸 （3）呼气宜浅，吸气宜深，尽可能使身体浮于水面，以等待救援 （4）不要将手上举或拼命挣扎，这样反而容易下沉
靠近溺水者	借助树枝、木棍、绳索或衣物等搭建与溺水者的桥梁
借助漂浮物	向溺水者抛漂浮物，可以是木材、救生圈、皮球、盖上盖子的空水瓶
借助船只	如果会使用船只，可以考虑借助船只救援
自救游回岸边	*会游泳者：* （1）会游泳者溺水可能是由于小腿腓肠肌痉挛，此时应平心静气，及时呼人援救 （2）自己将身体抱成一团，浮上水面 （3）深吸一口气，把面部浸入水中，将痉挛（抽筋）下肢的拇趾用力向前上方拉，使拇趾翘起来，持续用力，直到剧痛消失，痉挛也随即停止 （4）一次发作之后，同一部位可能再次痉挛，所以对疼痛处要充分按摩并慢慢游向岸边，上岸后最好再按摩和热敷患处 （5）如果手腕肌肉痉挛，可自行将手指上下屈伸，并采取仰面位，以两足游泳 *不会游泳者：* 不会游泳的溺水者可借助救生用具（如救生圈等）游回岸边
他救游回岸边	救护者应从背后接近，用一只手从背后抱住溺水者的头颈，另一只手抓住溺水者的手臂游向岸边

第三节 电击伤

电击伤俗称触电，是指一定量电流或电能量（静电）通过人体，引起的组织不同程度损伤或功能障碍，重者可发生心搏、呼吸骤停。

发现有人触电，该怎么办？

1. 确认现场环境安全。

2. 帮助触电者迅速脱离电源

（1）切断电源：拔除电源插头或拉下电源闸刀。

（2）挑开电线：用绝缘物或干燥木棒、竹竿、扁担等挑开电线。

（3）拉开触电者：穿胶鞋站在木凳或木板上，用干燥的绳子、围巾或干衣服等拧成条状套在触电者身上拉开触电者，不可直接接触触电者身体。

3. 呼喊触电者，观察胸廓起伏情况5～10秒，若无呼吸和反应，立即进行心肺复苏。

4. 触电者如有大面积烧伤，保护创面。

5. 迅速拨打"120"急救电话。

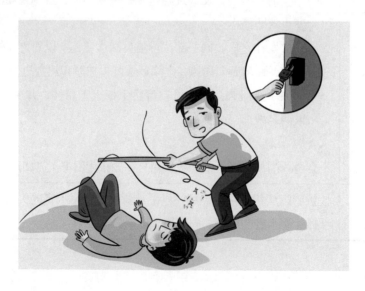

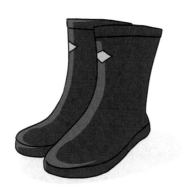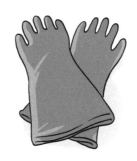

绝缘物

第四节　鼻出血与气道异物

一、鼻　出　血

遇到鼻腔出血时，用手指捏紧两侧鼻翼10～15分钟，同时以冷水袋或湿毛巾敷前额或后颈部，以减少出血，如出血量较多，请及时就医。

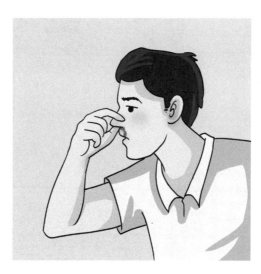

鼻出血

二、气道异物

（一）成人气道异物处理方法

1. 他救

发生气道异物后，首先需识别为不完全气道异物梗阻还是完全气道异物梗阻，对于前者需鼓励患者咳嗽，而对于后者，需立即使用海姆立克急救法急救。如患者清醒，急救者可以"前腿弓，后腿蹬"的姿势站稳，让患者身体略前倾，将双臂从患者腋下前伸环抱患者。一手握拳，另一手握住第一只手，第一只手拳贴在肚脐上方的腹部中央，然后突然用力收紧双臂，向上腹部内上方猛烈施压，致腹部下陷，每次猛压算1次动作，可重复进行，直至异物排出。

如患者意识丧失，使其取仰卧位于地面，立即开始心肺复苏。

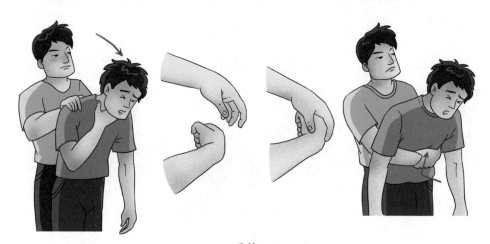

手势

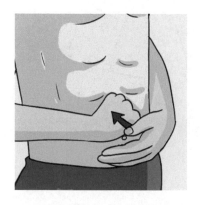

海姆立克腹部快速冲击法

2.自救

如果在紧急情况下，周围无一人在场，则可采用自救法。患者可左手握拳，右手从前方握住左手，左拳贴在肚脐上方的腹部中央，然后双臂发力，或以钝角物体快速向上冲压腹部，将异物排出，如腹部倚靠在椅背上快速冲击腹部。

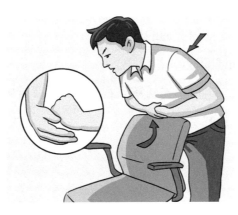

气道异物自救

（二）婴儿气道异物处理方法

将婴儿抱起，一手捏住颧骨两侧，手臂贴着婴儿的前胸，另一只手托住其后颈部，让其面部朝下，趴在救护人大腿上。在肩背上拍5次，并观察是否有异物排出。如果异物未排出，再将婴儿翻过来，将示指、中指并拢，在胸骨中下端按压5次。随时观察其口内有无异物排出，如异物排出，用手指将异物取出。以上动作应在婴儿头低于胸的情况下完成。如果无效，可重复上述动作。

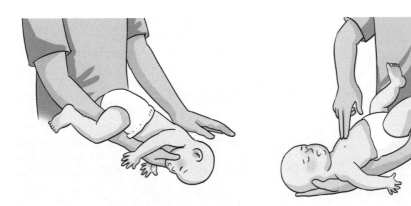

婴儿气道异物处理方法

第五节 交通事故

一、事故现场处理

（1）驾驶人应立即开启危险报警闪光灯。

（2）将车辆移至不妨碍交通的地点。

（3）在车后150m处设置警告标志。

（4）驾驶人和乘车人应迅速转移到右侧路肩上或者应急车道内。

（5）立即拨打"122"报警电话。

（6）保护现场，维持秩序。

二、现场救护

（一）心肺复苏

用5～10秒评估患者，如没有呼吸，则直接进行心肺复苏。

（二）控制出血

1. 直接加压法

用手掌或手指直接按在伤口上，并保持15分钟以上。

2. 高举法

将受伤的肢体抬高，使出血部位高于心脏，以减缓出血部位的血液流动。

3. 压迫止血法

当四肢有严重出血时，可压迫肢体的重要动脉。

（三）搬运伤员

1. 不要随意搬运伤员，特别是怀疑有颈椎、腰椎骨折的伤员。

2. 搬运前应先予以止血固定，可在现场寻找硬的树枝等，并用衣服给予包扎固定，然后再搬运。

3. 等待专业医务人员到场进行处理。

第六节　中　　毒

一、概　　述

中毒是指有毒化学物质通过一定的途径进入人体后，与人体相互作用，直接导致或者通过生物物理或生物化学反应，引起人体功能或结构发生改变，导致暂时性或持久性损害，甚至危及生命的疾病。毒物进入体内后是否发生中毒，取决于多种因素，如毒物的毒性、性状、进入体内的量和时间、患者的个体差异（如对毒物的敏感性及耐受性）等。

二、不同类型毒物中毒的应急处理方法

1. 清洁剂

如洗洁精、消毒剂、厨房清洁剂等，其所致中毒严重程度与摄入量相关，量少时主要为胃肠道刺激症状，量大时会引起胃肠道腐蚀、昏迷、抽搐等表现。

处理方法：立即至医院就诊，若昏迷，将患者头转向一侧，防止误吸。

2. 干燥剂

（1）硅啫喱：为半透明的小珠，不溶于水。若误服，不需要特殊处理，一般认为是无毒或低毒的。

（2）氧化钙：为白色或灰白色粉末，溶于水可形成氢氧化钙，是高度腐蚀性的。

（3）氯化钙：常用于衣柜内吸潮，为塑料包装，呈白色颗粒或絮状，在环境潮湿时溶解，具有高度腐蚀性。

处理方法：

（1）如果在误食30分钟内，可给予水、牛奶、蛋清等稀释和保护。

（2）不清楚毒物成分时，应带上毒物尽快就医。

3. 驱虫丸

市场上的驱虫丸常见成分是樟脑、萘、对二氯苯等，其中樟脑和萘毒性大。

处理方法： 带上毒物，尽快就医。

4. 酒精中毒

酒精可在胃和小肠内被快速吸收，饮酒5分钟后血中便可检测到酒精浓度。据有关资料统计，成人的平均酒精致死剂量为250～500g，酒精中毒严重程度与酒精摄入量相关，一般主要导致胃肠道刺激症状、轻度神经抑制症状等，严重时会引起昏迷、抽搐等表现。

处理方法：

（1）主要是预防呕吐引起的窒息，清醒者可饮用糖水。

（2）如果饮酒量大，患者反应较平常显著下降等，需立即就医。

第七节 动物致伤

一、概 述

不同类型动物通过不同途径对人体造成伤害，这种伤害具有较强的个体特异性。

二、不同类型动物咬伤的应急处理方法

1. 哺乳类动物咬伤

有咬痕或被撕裂的伤口，且伤口不规则，严重程度与伤口的大小、部位、污染程度等有关。

处理方法：

（1）简单清洗伤口，适当包扎、固定。不要在没有把握的情况下尝试自行拔出异物。

（2）由于动物（如猫和犬）牙齿带有很多细菌、病毒，除了常规的伤口处理外，最好前往附近的医院处理。

2. 蛇咬伤

处理方法：

（1）安抚患者，使其保持镇静，切勿惊慌、奔跑。

（2）应立即用柔软的绳或布带结扎在患肢近心端、伤口上方5cm左右，每隔15～30分钟放松1～2分钟，避免肢体组织缺血坏死，并对患肢进行固定。

（3）对于毒蛇咬伤，应急处理后，必须迅速将患者送往正规医院，按毒蛇咬伤进一步行规范急救治疗。

注意事项：所有蛇咬伤的伤病者均必须尽快送往医院。

3. 昆虫蜇伤或咬伤

主要表现为伤处局部灼痛、肿胀、发红、瘙痒，部分特殊昆虫甚至会导致哮喘发作、呼吸困难、昏迷。

处理方法：

（1）如被蜇伤后，发现皮肤上有毒毛、毒针尾端，可先用镊子将其拔掉。

（2）用流动的冷水仔细清洗蜇伤部位，之后冷敷。

（3）如果蜇伤部位局部红肿、疼痛明显，应尽快将蜇伤者送往就近医院处理。

注意事项：必须小心观察是否出现过敏性休克。

4. 水母蜇伤

蜇伤处红肿、疼痛、瘙痒，可伴有皮疹，严重者会出现呼吸困难、肌肉痉挛、昏迷等表现。

处理方法：

（1）被水母蜇伤应尽快离开水面。

（2）用海水冲洗伤口（不可用清水冲洗或用手接触触须），冷敷以减轻疼痛。

（3）严重蜇伤应立即寻求医疗救助。

第六章

常见急症救护

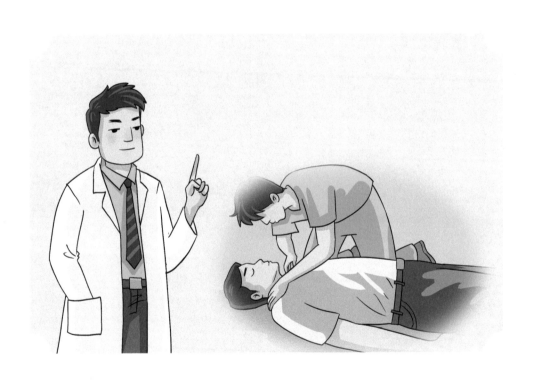

第一节　哮　　喘

一、概　　述

哮喘是一种慢性气道炎症性疾病。临床上，哮喘患者表现出反复发作的喘息、咳嗽、胸闷和呼吸急促。哮喘发作可能随时发生，但在夜间和早晨尤其常见。严重的哮喘发作可能危及生命，通常需要立即就医。

二、急救要点

（1）迅速为患者准备好药物及吸入装置，并帮助患者应用快速缓解症状的药物。

（2）帮助患者找到最舒适的体位，通常是坐位，身体微向前倾，靠在手肘或手臂上呼吸。

（3）留下一人来安慰和陪伴患者，避免多人站在患者身边，以免使患者更加焦虑。

（4）立即拨打"120"，需冷静而快速地将患者送往最近的医院。

第二节　胸　　痛

一、概　　述

胸痛是一种常见而又危急的临床症状，造成胸痛的原因复杂多样，一般为胸部疾病。常见引起胸痛的急症如下。

1. 冠心病

冠心病容易发生在"三高"（高血压、高血糖、高血脂）、长期吸烟、肥胖、有冠心病家族史的人群，冠心病胸痛通常表现为胸骨后疼痛，伴有出汗，持续5分钟以上，为憋闷样疼痛、喘不过气，像一颗大石头压在胸口。

2. 主动脉夹层

高血压是主动脉夹层的主要危险因素，血压控制不达标是其诱因。主动脉夹层疼痛常像刀割一样剧烈，难以忍受，有些人形容它为"平生最疼的一次"，持续时间较长，休息后不能缓解，也可能同时有后背痛、腹痛。

3. 肺栓塞

如果有肝肾功能不全、刚刚做过大手术、长期卧床少动、正在口服激素类药物等危险因素，就需要警惕肺栓塞的可能。除胸痛以外，肺栓塞通常还有呼吸困难、咯血、咳嗽咳痰等症状，严重时可能引起晕厥、休克等。

二、急救要点

胸痛是一种严重疾病，面对胸痛，须做到以下几点。

（1）对于胸痛应足够重视，切勿抱着"忍一忍"的心态，以免耽误病情。

（2）第一时间拨打"120"，不建议步行、坐车到医院就诊。

（3）让患者安静、平躺休息，等待救护人员到来。

（4）可用家用血压计测量血压、心率，做好记录。

（5）如果是冠心病高危人群，家中最好常备速效救心丸、硝酸甘油片、硝酸甘油喷雾等，胸痛出现时尽早使用。

第三节 脑 卒 中

一、概　述

脑卒中，也就是人们常说的"中风"，是一种急性脑血管疾病，包括出血性脑卒中（脑出血）和缺血性脑卒中（脑梗死），具有高致死率和高致残率等特点。数据显示，我国每年大约新增200万脑卒中患者，且呈现年轻化趋势，每年死于脑卒中的人数超过150万。脑卒中已成为我国首位致死原因，超过了所有癌症的总和。我国脑卒中高致死率、高致残率的主要原因是院前延误。

二、如何识别脑卒中

对脑卒中患者而言，时间就是生命。如何尽早识别脑卒中征兆？中国卒中学会中风120特别行动组提出了适合我国人群进行脑卒中快速识别的口诀——"中风120"，"1"即一张脸，患者面部是否出现口角歪斜、面部麻木、流涎等症状；"2"即两只胳膊，两只胳膊平抬时，是否出现一侧肢体无力或一侧肢体麻木的症状；"0"即聆听语言，是否出现吐字不清、言语困难或者不能言语等症状。如果发现上述任何突发症状，应迅速拨打"120"。

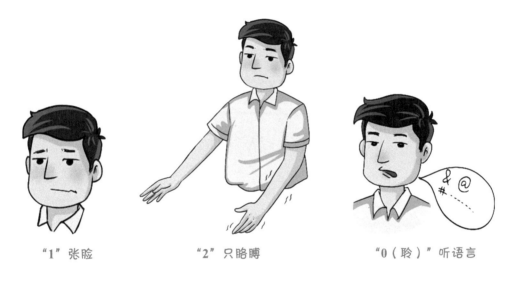

"1"张脸　　　　　"2"只胳膊　　　　　"0（聆）"听语言

三、到达医院后，医生会做什么

一般来说，医生会马上将患者安排在急诊科抢救室，连接心电监护，抽血化验、测血糖，并尽快行头颅CT检查。

若头颅CT检查提示没有脑出血，则会建议患者马上进行药物溶栓治疗甚至进一步行介入取栓术（可能需转至有相关条件的医院进一步治疗）；使用溶栓药物及行介入手术需要患者或家属签署相关同意书。

若头颅CT提示为脑出血，医生则会根据出血量的多少，收入院治疗或请神经外科会诊，行手术或介入治疗等。

在医院治疗过程中，维持生命体征稳定是治疗的基础，所以可能需要气管插管维持气道通畅、深静脉穿刺、使用血管活性药物、呼吸机辅助通气、插胃管、导尿等。

四、如何预防脑卒中

（1）控制血压是预防脑卒中的重点。高血压患者要按时服用降压药物，监测血压，饮食应清淡、有节制，戒烟限酒，适量运动，保持情绪平稳。

（2）防治动脉粥样硬化，关键在于防治高脂血症和肥胖。

（3）控制糖尿病和其他疾病如心脏病、脉管炎等。

（4）注意气象因素的影响：季节与气候变化会使高血压患者情绪不稳、血压波动，诱发脑卒中，这时更要预防脑卒中的发生。

第四节　高　血　压

一、概　　述

成年人非同日 3 次血压超过 140/90mmHg 即可诊断为高血压。中国成年人高血压患病率高达 25.2%，即约 4 个人中就有 1 人患高血压。

二、高血压的危害

高血压属于慢性病，是导致脑卒中、冠心病和肾衰竭最重要的危险因素。据统计，全国每年有 200 万人死于与高血压有关的疾病，并且 60% 以上的冠心病患者、80% 以上的脑梗死患者、90% 的脑出血患者都有高血压病史。可以说，高血压是人类健康的"隐形杀手"。

三、高血压的表现

高血压通常没有较为明显的症状，常见的临床症状有头痛、头晕、注意力不集中、记忆力减退、肢体麻木、夜尿增多、心悸、胸闷、乏力等。

四、高血压常见问题解答

1. 长期服用降压药是否会上瘾

降压药不是成瘾药物，不会上瘾。患者应在医生指导下规范、合理口服降压药治疗，这样既不会对身体造成损害，也有助于控制好血压。

2. 血压控制达标后能否停药

有高血压患者认为，服用降压药将血压降至正常，便意味着高血压已治好，就可以停药。殊不知，停药后血压可能会再次升高，而间歇用药易引起血压波动，会带来更大的危害。高血压患者应在医生指导下，小心地逐渐调整药物的剂量和种类以适合自身情况，不可自行停药或增减药量。

3. 保健品能否替代降压药

有些患者认为西药副作用大，不愿意长期服用，又听闻某些保健品能降血压，于是盲目依赖保健品。实际上，保健品降压效果并不可靠，虽然有些保健品有一定的辅助降压作用，但不能仅依靠保健品进行降压治疗，因此保健品并不能替代降压药。

4. 单纯食疗能否降血压

饮食是治疗高血压的基础，可通过饮食干预延缓血压进一步升高，但达不到控制血压的目的。因此，大多数情况下，不能单纯通过食疗降血压。

5. 能否自行去药店购买与其他高血压患者相同的降压药服用

降压方案存在个体差异，不应依据他人的用药方案用药。患者应在医生指导下对血压进行动态监测，根据血压水平及时调整用药。

6. 血压突然升高怎么办

在某些诱因作用下，血压突然和显著升高（一般超过180/120mmHg），若同时伴有进行性心、脑、肾等重要靶器官功能急性损害，临床称为高血压急症；若不伴靶器官功能损害，则称为高血压亚急症。

这两种情况均是有高度危险性的心血管急危重症，须及时、有效治疗。患者应即刻到医院就诊，接受专科治疗，避免发生严重并发症。

第五节 休 克

一、概 述

休克是机体遭受严重致病因素侵袭后，由于有效循环血量急剧减少，组织血流灌注广泛、持续、显著减少，致全身微循环功能不良、生命重要器官严重功能障碍的综合征。

二、临床表现

休克的临床表现有血压降低、少尿甚至无尿、皮肤湿冷、肢体皮肤呈花斑样改变、意识障碍等。

三、病 因

休克的病因包括心源性因素、过敏性因素、感染性因素、肺栓塞等。

休克是临床上常见的紧急且威胁患者生命的情况，死亡率较高，临床表现出现较晚，一旦出现低血压，病情可能已经恶化，必须马上进行救治。在休克早期进行有效干预，控制引起休克的原发病因，遏止病情发展，有助于改善患者预后。

第六节 糖 尿 病

一、概 述

糖尿病是一组因胰岛素绝对和相对分泌不足和（或）胰岛素利用障碍引起的碳水化合物、蛋白质、脂肪代谢紊乱性疾病，以高血糖为主要标志。

人体能够通过激素调节和神经调节这两大调节系统使血糖的来源与去路保持动态平衡，使血糖维持在一定水平。然而，在遗传因素（如有糖尿病家族史）与环境因素（如不合理膳食、肥胖等）的共同作用下，两大调节系统发生紊乱，就会出现血糖水平的升高（高血糖急症）或降低（低血糖急症）。

二、临 床 表 现

1. 高血糖急症的表现

多饮、多食、多尿、体重减轻、视物模糊、疲倦嗜睡等。

2. 低血糖急症的表现

饥饿感、头晕、心慌、手抖、出冷汗、大汗淋漓，严重时出现意识障碍、昏迷甚至死亡。

3. 糖尿病并发症

糖尿病并发症包括视网膜病变、脑卒中、急性心肌梗死、动脉粥样硬化、周围神经病变及糖尿病肾病等。

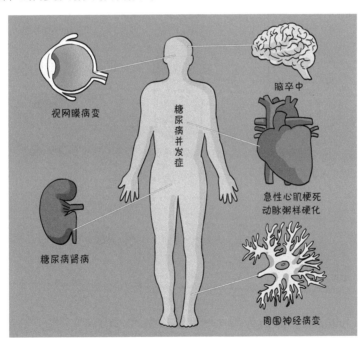

三、急救处理措施

1. 高血糖急症的处理方法

因患者需要胰岛素或其他药物治疗，出现高血糖急症时应立即将其送往医院进行降血糖治疗，并密切监测血糖变化。若患者昏迷，将其送往医院的同时，应让患者平躺，头偏向一侧，防止窒息。

2. 低血糖急症的处理方法

（1）若患者清醒，可扶患者坐下或躺下；若患者昏迷，应立即将其送往医院进行治疗。

（2）患者可进食时，给予含15g糖的快速升糖食物，在情况稳定时及时就医，若情况并无改善，检查患者有无其他致昏迷原因，并尽早送往医院治疗。

（3）保持患者气道通畅，检查患者呼吸、脉搏及反应程度。

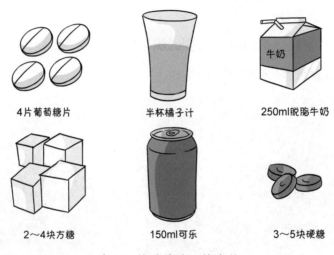

4片葡萄糖片　　　　半杯橘子汁　　　　250ml脱脂牛奶

2～4块方糖　　　　150ml可乐　　　　3～5块硬糖

含 15g 糖的快速升糖食物

第七节 癫 痫

一、概 述

癫痫（epilepsy）即俗称的"羊角风"或"羊癫风"，是大脑神经元突发性异常放电，导致短暂的大脑功能障碍的一种慢性疾病。

二、急救处理措施

（1）确保患者癫痫发作时处于安全状态，把患者搬离高处、危处，保证患者身边没有尖锐物体（包括眼镜）；如果患者此时尚未倒地，则马上扶住患者，确保患者平衡，再缓慢帮助患者处于卧位。这一操作的目的是给患者提供一个安全的空间，避免二次损伤，临床上有不少患者因癫痫发作倒地导致脑出血，或者肢体抽动打翻热水导致烫伤。

（2）确保患者呼吸道通畅。患者躺下后，将其翻转至侧卧位，如果不方便，可以将患者头转向一侧。因为有的患者发作时会出现口吐白沫的症状，这一操作可以有效避免分泌物误吸入气管，还能防止舌根后坠、堵塞气道。口鼻腔分泌物或者异物误吸短时间内可引起窒息，或者发作期间症状不明显，后期出现吸入性肺炎，故切勿忽视。

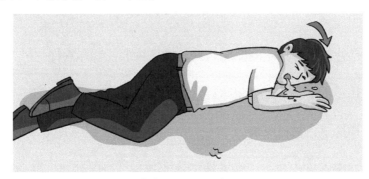

将患者转至侧卧位

（3）如患者打领带或者衣服太紧，需松开领带，酌情解开或脱掉紧身衣物以利于患者呼吸。一般情况下癫痫发作有自限性，发作几分钟会自行终止，但是常见的强直-阵挛性发作（即最常见的"大发作"）一般发作时间可超过5分钟，进入癫痫持续状态，需要药物干预终止发作。

注意事项：

（1）按压人中并不能终止癫痫发作。

（2）癫痫发作时，勿往患者口中塞各种物体，以免引起窒息。

（3）患者清醒前不要试图喂水，以免引起误吸。

（4）抽搐时，不要用力按压患者肢体，以免造成骨折或扭伤。

第八节　中　暑

一、概　述

中暑是指在温度或湿度较高、不透风的环境下，因体温调节中枢功能障碍或汗腺功能衰竭，以及水、电解质丢失过多，从而发生的以中枢神经和（或）心血管功能障碍为主要表现的急性疾病。可表现为眩晕、高热（体温39.1～41.0℃）、少汗、呕吐、心悸、肢体抽搐等。

二、急救处理措施

移：迅速将患者移至阴凉通风处，垫高头部，解开衣物。

敷：用冷毛巾敷头部或将冰袋置于头部、腋窝、大腿根部。

擦：用冷毛巾擦拭全身。

浸：对于重度中暑者，将其置于冷水浸泡，同时按摩四肢皮肤，促进血液循环，加速散热。

第九节　发　热

一、概　述

发热指在致热原作用下，使体温调节中枢的调定点上移而引起调节性体温升高。而发热程度（以口温为标准，腋温低于口温0.3～0.5℃）分为低热：37.3～38.0℃；中热：38.1～39.0℃；高热：39.1～41.0℃；超高热：41.0℃以上。

二、临床表现

发热可分为体温上升期、高热持续期、体温下降期，不同的时期有不同的症状。体温上升期患者通常表现为疲劳无力，伴随一定程度的四肢肌肉酸痛，或皮肤干燥苍白，这时因产热大于散热，体温持续上升。高热持续期，患者体温会维持在较高水平，伴皮肤潮红和灼热，以及心率、呼吸加快。体温下降期主要表现为大量出汗和皮肤温度降低。

三、急救处理措施

（1）如有高热惊厥前趋症状，应将牙垫置于上下牙齿之间，防止咬伤舌头。

（2）松开衣服领口，把头部偏向一侧，方便分泌物流出。

（3）及时拨打"120"。

第七章

灾难逃生与救护

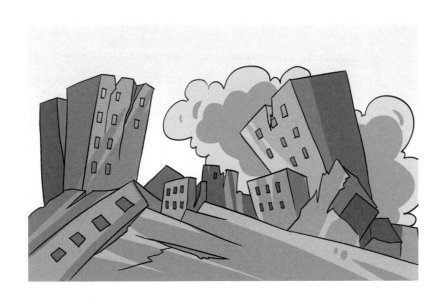

自然灾害具有突发性，人们往往难以预料和防范，因此伤害程度大。在灾害来临之前应掌握灾害防范相关知识，学习初级自救互救本领，做好心理准备。一旦灾害来临，会逃生、会救护能减轻灾害带来的损失。本章着重介绍几种常见灾害的逃生和救护知识。

第一节　地　震

一、概　述

地震在自然灾害中属于受灾面积广、破坏性强、死伤人数多的地质灾害，往往会在瞬间给人类和社会造成巨大损失。

地震造成人员伤亡的原因有建筑物倒塌、煤气泄漏、触电、溺水和火灾等，其中最常见的是建筑物倒塌。

在保证救护人员安全的前提下，现场应遵循先近后远、先抢后救的原则，开展对震区人员的搜索、脱险、救护医疗一体化的大救援。

二、现场救护要点

（1）对于埋在瓦砾中的幸存者，先建立通风孔道，以防窒息；挖出后应立即清除伤病员口鼻异物和压在其头面部、胸腹部的泥土，对眼睛予以避光保护。检查伤病员，判断其意识、呼吸、循环体征。

（2）从缝隙中缓慢将伤病员救出时，应保持脊柱呈中立位，以免伤及脊髓。

（3）救出伤病员后，即刻检查其伤情，遇神志不清、大出血等急危重症者应优先救护，对外伤、出血给予包扎、止血，骨折予以固定，对于脊柱骨折者要正确搬运。

（4）因恐惧心理，原有心脏病、高血压者病情可加重、复发，引起猝死，对此类伤病员要特别关注。

（5）身处危险环境中的自救方法

1）设法避开身体上方不结实的倒塌物、悬挂物或其他危险物，用砖石、木棍等支撑残垣断壁，以防余震时再被埋压。

2）搬开身边可搬动的碎砖瓦等杂物，扩大活动空间。

3）不要随便动用室内设施，包括电源、水源等，不要使用明火。

4）不要大喊大叫，应保存体力，用敲击的方法求救。

5）闻到煤气及异味时，要用湿衣物捂住口鼻。

6）保护和节约使用饮用水、食物。

三、各种场所的避震

躲避原则：就近选择可形成三角空间的地方躲避；逃离危险场所；避开易发生灾害处；切断危险源；避免人为事故。

（一）室内避震

迅速躲在坚固家具附近或内墙墙根、墙角等易形成三角空间的地方。如果离厨房、卫生间、储藏室等空间小的地方很近，可以迅速躲到里面。不要跳楼，不要站在窗边及靠近阳台的墙边，更不要到阳台上。

（二）学校避震

（1）在操场或室外时，可原地不动蹲下，双手保护头部，注意避开高大建筑物或危险物。不要回到教室。

（2）如果在室内，当老师给出避险信号时，应立即用手保护头及眼部，迅速躲到桌子下面。逃生时千万不要跳楼，也不要站在窗外或到阳台去。

（3）震后应当有组织地撤离，避免人员密集。

（三）公共场所避震

听从现场工作人员的指挥，就近在牢固物旁蹲伏。有序撤离，不要慌乱；避免拥挤，避开人流；不要乘坐电梯，也不要在楼梯间停留。在体育场馆、影剧院内，就地蹲下或趴在排椅旁，注意避开悬挂物，用书包等保护头部。在商场、书店、展览馆、地铁站等地，选择结实的柜台、商品（如低矮的家具等）或柱子边，以及内墙角等处就地蹲下，用手或其他东西保护头部。在行驶的电车、汽车内，要抓牢扶手，降低重心，躲在座位附近。

（四）户外避震

就地选择开阔地蹲下或趴下，以免跌倒，不要乱跑，避开人多的地方；不要随便返回室内。避开高大建筑物，特别是有玻璃幕墙的建筑；避开过街桥、立交桥、高烟囱、水塔等；避开危险物，如变压器、电线杆、路灯、广告牌等；避开其他危险场所，如狭窄的街道、危旧房屋、危墙、女儿墙、高门脸、雨篷下及砖瓦木料等物的堆放处；避开公路、铁路。

第二节　火　　灾

一、概　　述

火灾是指在时间或空间上失去控制的燃烧所造成的灾害，可对人身和财产造成一定损害。

二、现场救护要点

1. 不入险地，不贪财物

生命是最重要的，不要因为害羞或顾及贵重物品，而把宝贵的逃生时间浪费在穿衣或寻找、拿走贵重物品上。

2. 简易防护，不可缺少

家中、公司等应备有防烟面罩，也可用毛巾、口罩蒙鼻，用水浇身，匍匐前进。因为烟气较空气轻而飘于上部，贴近地面逃离是避免烟气吸入的最佳方法。

3. 缓降逃生，滑绳自救

千万不要盲目跳楼，可利用疏散楼梯、阳台、落水管等进行逃生自救，也可用身边的绳索、床单、窗帘、衣服自制简易救生绳*，并用水打湿，紧拴在窗框、暖气管、铁栏杆等固定物上，用毛巾、布条等保护手心、顺绳滑下，或下到未着火的楼层脱离险境。

4. 当机立断，快速撤离

受到火势威胁时，要当机立断披上浸湿的衣物、被褥等向安全出口方向逃生，千万不要盲目地跟从人流相互拥挤、乱冲乱撞。撤离时，要注意朝明亮处或外面空旷地逃生。当火势不大时要尽量往楼层下面跑，若通道被烟火封阻，则应背向烟火方向，逃到天台、阳台处。

5. 善用通道，莫入电梯

遇火灾不可乘坐电梯或扶梯，要向安全出口方向逃生。

6. 大火袭来，固守待援

大火袭来，假如用手摸房门已感发烫，不要开门，若此时开门，火焰和浓烟将扑来。此时可关紧门窗，用湿毛巾、湿布塞堵门缝，或用水浸湿棉被，蒙上门窗，防止烟火渗入，等待救援人员到来。

7. 火已烧身，切勿惊跑

身上着火，千万不要奔跑，可就地打滚或用厚重的衣物压灭火苗。

8. 发出信号，寻求救援

若所有逃生线路均被大火封锁，要立即退回室内，用打手电筒、挥舞衣物、呼叫等方式向外发送求救信号，引起救援人员的注意。

9. 熟悉环境，暗记出口

无论是居家，还是到学校、商场等公共场所时，务必留心疏散通道、安全出口及楼梯方位等，当大火燃起、浓烟密布时，便可以摸清道路，尽快逃离现场。

---

* 自制简易救生绳时，要注意牢固性和长度等问题，以避免可能的风险。

第三节　水　　灾

一、概　述

水灾是指由于特大暴雨或沿海地区的特大高潮等，河流、海洋、湖泊等水体上涨超过一定水位，致使洪水地区的人、房屋、耕地、工厂等遭到损害，威胁有关地区的安全，对人类社会造成灾害的事件。

二、现场救护要点

（1）洪水到来时，首先应迅速登上牢固的高层建筑避险，之后与救援部门取得联系，同时注意收集木盆、木桶、木块等漂浮材料作为救护设备，可扎制木排以备急需。

（2）避难所一般应选在距家最近、地势较高、交通较为方便处，最好有水源设施，卫生条件较好。在城市中大多是高层建筑的平坦楼顶，有牢固楼房的学校、医院，以及地势高的公园等。

（3）若时间允许，做好准备工作。用木盆等盛水工具储备干净的饮用水；备好医药、取火物品等；将衣被等御寒物品放至高处保存；不便携带的贵重物品做防水捆扎后埋入地下或者放于高处；票款、首饰等可缝在衣物中。

（4）保存好各种尚能使用的通信设施，与外界保持良好的通信、交通联系。

（5）如洪水继续上涨，暂避的地方已难自保，则要充分利用准备好的逃生器材逃生，或迅速找一些漂浮材料扎成筏逃生。

（6）若已被洪水包围，要设法尽快与当地防汛部门取得联系，报告自己的方位和险情，积极寻求救援。注意：千万不要游泳逃生，不可攀爬带电的电线杆、铁塔，也不要爬到泥坯房的屋顶，发现高压线、铁塔倾斜或者电线断头下垂时，一定要迅速远避。

（7）若已被卷入洪水中，一定要尽可能抓住固定的或能漂浮的物体，寻找机会逃生。

（8）在山区，如果连降大雨，容易暴发山洪。应该注意避免过河，以防被山洪冲走，还要注意防止山体滑坡、滚石、泥石流的伤害。

（9）洪水过后，要做好各项卫生防疫工作，预防疫病的流行。

第四节 雷 击

一、概 述

雷击的接触点通常是电流进出人体的点，因此大多发生在头部、颈部或肩部。伤员表现为皮肤被烧焦、鼓膜或内脏被震裂、心室颤动、心脏停搏、呼吸肌麻痹。被雷击后，若心搏并无停止迹象，预后多较好，因此当多人被雷击时，应先抢救状似死亡的患者，实时施予心肺复苏术，使心脏和脑很快得到氧气，急救得当可以拯救生命，并将伤害降到最低。

二、现场救护要点

1. 雷击发生关键在于预防

现代科技已可以预知雷雨的发生，因此采取一些措施可以预防雷击带来的危害。

（1）雷雨天不宜在室外走动或在大树下避雨，要拿掉身上的金属物，蹲下防雷击。

（2）打雷时远离电灯、电源，不靠近柱和墙壁，防止引起感应电。

（3）关好门窗、家电，关电门。

（4）在室外者如感到头发竖立、皮肤刺痛、肌肉发抖，即可能有将被闪电击中的危险，应立即蹲下，并尽量减少与地面的接触面积，可避免雷击。切勿躺在地上，潮湿的地面尤其危险。通过以上这些措施可以有效避免雷击伤，或将伤害降到最低程度。

2. 雷击一般会导致心·搏骤停

应立刻评估患者，如5～10秒未发现胸廓起伏，应立即开始心肺复苏，并拨打"120"急救电话。

第五节　垂直电梯遇险

一、概　　述

电梯故障通常会给受困者的心理造成恐慌，遇到此种情况切不可轻举妄动，因为此时电梯内反而是安全的。

二、现场救护要点

（1）不论有几层楼，迅速按下每层楼的按键，当紧急电源启动时，电梯可以马上停止继续下坠。

（2）电梯下坠时整个背部和头部紧贴电梯内墙，使其呈一条直线，利用电梯墙壁保护脊椎。

（3）如果电梯内有扶手，最好紧握扶手以固定位置，防止因重心不稳而跌伤。如果电梯内没有扶手，用手抱颈部，避免颈部受伤。

（4）膝盖呈弯曲姿势，因为韧带是人体最有弹性的一个组织，可通过膝盖弯曲来承受重击压力。

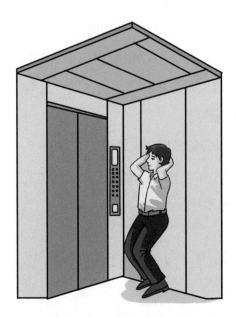

电梯下坠时保护自己的最佳姿势

切忌以下行为：

（1）切忌采取过激行为，如在电梯内乱蹦乱跳。

（2）切忌强行扒门爬出，以防电梯突然启动。

第六节　野外遇险

一、概　　述

在野外时，灾难或危急状况可能不期而至，因此有必要掌握野外求救的技巧。当在野外身陷险境时，可利用移动电话和周围的资源发出求救信号。使求救的目标增大或与周围环境明显区分，能够更有效地传达求救信号，以便在遇险时尽快获救。

二、野外遇险求救信号

野外遇险时可通过下列方法向地面、海上和空中发出求救信号，重复三次以寻求帮助。

（一）视觉信号

1. 地空联络符号

SOS（求救）是国际通用的紧急求救信号，也可以在空旷处摆放 HELP（帮助）、SEND（送出）、DOCTOR（医生）、INJURY（受伤）、TRAPPED（发射）、LOST（迷失）、WATER（水）等字样。寻找比较开阔的草地、雪地、海滩制作地面标志，如把青草割成一定标志图案，或在雪地上踩出求救标志，也可用树枝、海草等拼成求救标志和信号，与空中取得联络。

2. 强光电筒

强光电筒分为强光、弱光、频闪三个模式，频闪模式通常用于求救。

3. 烟火信号

国际通用烟火求救信号是三堆呈等边三角形的火堆。白天，烟雾是良好定位器，在火堆上添加些绿草、树叶、苔藓和蕨类植物会产生浓烟，潮湿的草席、坐垫则可熏烧较长时间。黑色烟雾在雪地或沙漠中最醒目，橡胶和汽油可产生黑烟。

4. 反光信号

利用阳光和一面反射镜（如玻璃、金属片等）即可射出信号光，持续反射将规律性地产生一条长线和一个圆点，这是莫尔斯码的一种。即使不懂莫尔斯码，随意反照，也能引人注目。

5. 体示信号

站在高处，双手大幅度挥舞与周围环境颜色反差较大的衣物，表达遇险的意思。

6. 旗语信号

将一面旗子或一块色泽明艳的布料系在木棒上，持棒运动：左侧长划，右侧短划，做"8"字形运动。

（二）听觉信号

大声呼喊或用木棒敲打树干、管道，救生哨的作用会更明显，救生哨的尖锐哨声能引起搜救人员注意，记住哨声一定要有节奏，即三短、三长、三短，间隔1分钟之后再重复。

（三）方向指示标

一路上要不断留下指示标，这有助于搜救人员寻找你的行动路径。

（1）将岩石或碎石片摆成箭头形。

（2）将棍棒支撑在树杈间，顶部指着行动的方向。

（3）在草的中上部系结，使其顶端弯曲指示行动方向。

（4）用小石块垒成一个大石堆，在边上再放一小石块指向行动方向。

（5）用一个深刻于树干的箭头形凹槽表示行动方向。

（6）两根交叉的木棒或石头意味着此路不通。

（7）用三块岩石、木棒或灌木丛传达危险或紧急信号。

三、救援电话号码

公安报警电话：**110**。

消防报警电话：**119**。

急救电话：**120**。

交通事故报警电话：**122**，**12122**（高速公路报警救援电话）。

水上救援电话：**12395**。

城建服务热线（公共交通、供水、燃气、供热、违章建筑等问题）：**12319**。

供电服务热线：**95598**。

天气预报热线：**12121**。

红十字会急救电话：**999**。

第八章

心理急救

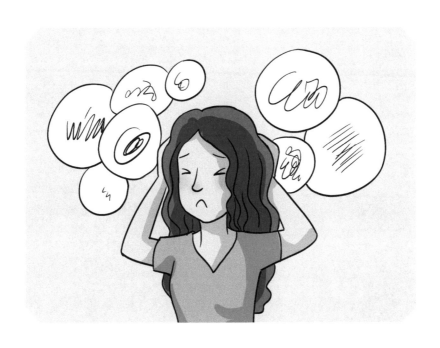

一、概　述

急救不应仅针对身体，心理也同样重要，如果心理创伤得不到解决，可能造成难以逾越的心理障碍。

二、情感创伤急救箱组成

1. 急救"药品"

水果、茶、家乡菜、绿植、鲜花、香水、音乐等。

2. 急救"器械"

玩偶、画具、笔墨纸砚、游泳装备、羽毛球、远足装备等。

3. 急救场地

室内、户外。

4. 急救人员

自己或信任的老师、朋友、辅导员、心理卫生专业人士、心理咨询师、专业心理医生等。

三、急救具体步骤

1. 珍视自己

记住自己是世界上独一无二的，生命珍贵。人的一生可能会经历情绪低落、挫败感、失败、内疚、沮丧、被拒绝、分离、丧失、焦虑、失望、自卑、孤独、社交恐惧、愤怒、抑郁、无助、失恋、失业、遭遇车祸、亲人离世等痛苦，每个人都会与情感创伤不期而遇。要清楚我们体验到的一切痛苦是可以被理解的，也是合理的。

2. 掌握情感创伤急救技能

情感创伤如同身体创伤，需要自行处置或去医院治疗。可寻求一些治疗方案来处理、抚慰受伤的情绪，振作精神，战胜挫折，打破负能量循环。

3. 选择坚强

相信自己的情感免疫系统能改变糟糕情绪，暗示自己是个幸运的人，经常性地进行情绪保健，保持精神健康，有信心克服困难和走出困境。

4. 搁置问题，以逸待劳

可以通过洗热水澡、睡觉休息，养精蓄锐。

5. 寻找、培养乐趣

如画画、写毛笔字、摄影、篆刻、拼装玩具等，或外出看电影，听相声，做运动，欣赏绿植、鲜花、音乐等，或者家养小动物、栽培农作物、花草盆景等。

6. 居家休养

从独处的住所回到家乡，看望父母，和父母一起劳动，收拾家居环境。照顾身体衰老的长辈，抚育子女等。烹饪食物，烘焙，向亲人朋友倾诉或静静陪伴。

7. 旅行

在旅行中可感受和体验大自然，欣赏风景，或认识新的朋友。

第九章

妊娠期健康

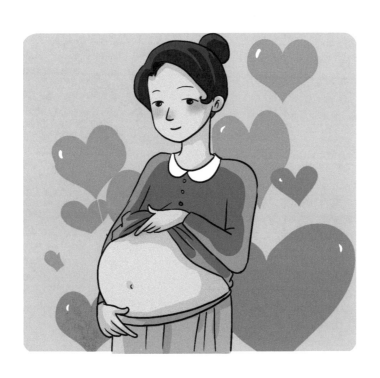

一、概　　述

妊娠期保健即通过积极的预防、普查、监护和保健措施，做好妊娠各期保健，以减少和控制某些疾病及遗传病的发生，降低孕产妇死亡率，促进妇女身心健康。

二、确 认 妊 娠

停经是妊娠的一个重要信息，但是停经不一定意味着妊娠，要到正规医院进行检查后方可确诊。

三、预产期与妊娠期计算

1. 推算预产期

明确末次月经的日期，推算预产期。计算方法：末次月经第一日起，月份减3或加9，日期加7；如为阴历，月份仍减3或加9，但日期加15。实际分娩日期与推算的预产期可以相差1～2周。

2. 妊娠分期

妊娠期从末次月经第一日开始计算，约为280日（40周）。临床上分为3个时期：妊娠开始到妊娠12周末为早期妊娠，第13～27周末为中期妊娠，第28周及其后的阶段称为晚期妊娠。

四、妊娠期常见表现

1. 早期妊娠的表现

早期妊娠可出现恶心呕吐、尿频尿急、白带增多等症状，如出现阴道出血，要及时到医院就诊。

2. 中、晚期妊娠的表现

中、晚期妊娠可出现水肿，下肢、外阴静脉曲张，便秘，痔疮，腰背痛，下肢痉挛，仰卧位低血压，失眠，贫血等症状。

五、妊娠期生活指导

1. 妊娠前3个月及末3个月

均应避免性生活，以防流产、早产及感染等情况的发生。

2. 妊娠期自我监护

（1）胎心音和胎动计数是孕妇自我监护胎儿宫内情况的重要手段。指导孕妇或家属正确听胎心音并做记录，不仅有助于了解胎儿宫内发育情况，而且可以促进家庭成员之间的亲情关系。

（2）一般孕妇在妊娠20周开始自觉胎动，胎动通常在夜间和下午较为活跃。孕妇可于每日早、中、晚各数1小时胎动，每小时胎动数应不少于3次，12小时内胎动数累计不得少于10次。

3. 药物的使用

许多药物可通过胎盘进入胚胎内而影响胚胎发育，尤其在妊娠最初2个月，此时是胚胎器官发育、形成时期，用药更应注意。

孕妇合理用药原则：能用一种药时，避免联合用药；选用疗效明确的药物，避免用尚难确定对胎儿是否有不良反应的药物；能用小剂量药物时，避免用大剂量药物；严格掌握用药剂量和持续时间，注意及时停药。若病情需要，选用了对胚胎、胎儿有害的致畸药物，应先终止妊娠，然后用药。

4. 其他

如乘坐汽车时，应避免安全带直接勒住腹部，应绑在大腿根部（腹股沟）的位置。

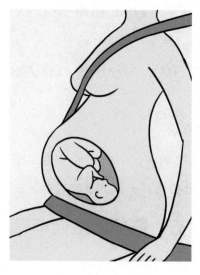

安全带正确位置

六、妊娠期需立即就诊的情况

孕妇出现下列症状应立即就诊：呕吐严重或妊娠3个月后仍持续呕吐，头痛、眼花，胸闷、心悸、气短，下肢明显凹陷性水肿或休息后不能缓解，寒战发热，腹部疼痛，胎动异常，阴道出血，胎膜早破，阴道排液，胎动计数突然减少等。

1. 胎动异常

妊娠28周后，凡12小时内胎动数累计少于10次或逐日下降大于50%而不能恢复者，提示胎儿有宫内缺氧可能，应及时就诊，以便进一步诊断并处理。

2. 阴道出血

妊娠早期若出现阴道鲜红色出血伴或不伴疼痛，可能与先兆流产、宫颈病变、宫外孕或葡萄胎等有关，应及时就医。

妊娠中、晚期阴道出血有可能是前置胎盘和胎盘早剥导致，如孕妇有阴道出血，不论量多少都应提高警惕，并及时到医院就诊。

3. 胎膜早破

临产前胎膜破裂称为胎膜早破，表现为孕妇突感从阴道流出较多的液体。一旦发生胎膜早破，孕妇应取平卧位，由家属送往医院，以防脐带脱垂而危及胎儿生命。

七、识别先兆临产

分娩发动前，一般会出现一些预示临产的症状，如不规律宫缩、胎儿下降感及阴道出现少量血性分泌物（俗称见红），称为先兆临产。经产妇出现不规律宫缩即可到医院就诊，预防急产。

开始规律宫缩（间歇5～6分钟，持续30秒或以上），且逐渐增强，同时伴随进行性宫颈管消失、宫口扩张和胎先露部下降，称为临产，此时应尽快到医院就诊。

八、院外紧急分娩

随着三孩政策的实施,孕妇在院外紧急分娩的情况有可能增加,若孕妇不能被及时送往医院分娩,须就地紧急分娩时,可采取下列处理步骤。

1. 孕妇确认分娩征兆

如果孕妇突然感到不由自主地想用力,有大便感,并且感觉越来越强烈,甚至开始觉得胎儿要往下掉,说明即将要分娩。

2. 立即求助

孕妇及其家属应立即拨打"120"急救电话,并就地向有关工作人员求助。

3. 深呼吸

当宫缩开始时,嘱孕妇用鼻深深吸气,然后再用口慢慢吐气,指导孕妇不要过早屏气用力。

4. 因地制宜

救助者应观察现场环境,尽快安置孕妇到就近、安全和隐蔽的场所,临时搭建"产床"。若有床,则铺一层干净的床单,在孕妇臀部下垫护理垫或干净的毛巾;若无床,则在相对干净的地面铺多件清洁的衣物和毛巾。

5. 平卧

救助者让孕妇仰卧、屈膝,脱去干扰分娩的衣物,用衣服或其他盖物遮盖住孕妇身体,随时注意阴道口胎头情况。

6. 清洁消毒

如果时间允许,用清洁剂或肥皂水清洗孕妇会阴部,接生者的双手也应进行清洗和消毒,有条件时尽量戴上手套(现场可找替代物)。

7. 胎头未露

若阴道口未见胎头,指导孕妇取左侧卧位,调整呼吸,不用力。

8. 胎头已露

若阴道口见胎儿毛发或部分头部,且胎头快速向外娩出,指导孕妇打开双腿,大口哈气,不要用力,准备接生。

9. 帮助娩出胎头

胎头娩出过程中，让孕妇快速哈气，接生者左手手掌扶住胎头控制胎头娩出速度，右手持干净的软垫（或替代物）向上托住会阴（肛门上方），让胎头慢慢滑出阴道。胎头娩出后，左手从胎儿下颌轻轻向上挤压，右手从鼻根轻轻向下挤压，以挤出胎儿口鼻腔内的黏液和羊水。

10. 娩肩

等待一次宫缩后，向下轻压胎儿颈部娩出前肩，然后用左手向上托住胎儿颈部，娩出后肩，不要强拉，此过程仍然需要右手向上托住保护会阴以预防会阴严重撕裂；两侧肩膀露出后，托住新生儿身体使其慢慢娩出，妥善接稳，防止坠地。

11. 新生儿娩出后

用一块干净纱布拭抹新生儿口鼻内的黏液或污血，并立即擦干其身体，通常新生儿在出生1分钟内会自行啼哭，如未哭应摩擦其背部或拍打足部刺激其啼哭，新生儿大声啼哭表示气道通畅。

12. 注意脐带处理

新生儿啼哭后，在距离新生儿脐带根部15cm和20cm处分别用干净的夹子或绳子扎紧，切记不可任意剪断脐带。

13. 皮肤接触

处理完毕后，接生者将新生儿连接着脐带，腹部朝下趴在产妇腹部上，头偏向一侧，接着用干净的毛巾和衣物盖好新生儿和产妇。

14. 等待胎盘娩出

通常新生儿出生5～15分钟后，胎盘便可以自然娩出，不要用力强行牵拉胎盘。如阴道少量出血，可适当牵拉脐带以娩出胎盘。

15. 胎盘处置

胎盘娩出后，应连接着脐带妥善放置在一边，不可剪断丢弃。

16. 按摩子宫

轻轻按摩肚脐周围子宫的上方位置，促使子宫收缩变硬，以减少出血。

17. 产后护理

卧床休息，并注意保暖，等待医务人员到达。

注意事项：为避免危险情况的发生，在临近分娩时，最好不要让孕妇单独待在家中。此外，临近预产期，应提前准备好入院手续和待产用品，查清楚医院行车路线，熟悉入院流程。

第十章
感染控制与预防措施

一、概　　述

急救人员在进行急救的同时应注意个人安全防护，采取正确而有效的预防及安全措施，避免与患者发生交叉感染。此外，需在标准预防的基础上正确认识疾病的传播途径，增加正确的个人防护。感染性疾病的传播途径可分为空气传播、飞沫传播及接触传播。病原体可以通过血液、体液、分泌物、排泄物、呕吐物等进行传播，掌握感染性疾病传播途径及防护要点相关知识至关重要。

二、基本防护知识

1. 标准预防的概念

标准预防是指认为患者的血液、体液、分泌物（不包括汗液）、排泄物等均具有传染性，接触时需进行自我保护，不论是否有明显的血迹污染或是否接触非完整的皮肤与黏膜，接触上述物质者必须采取防护措施。

2. 标准预防措施

（1）救护人员救护患者过程中可能沾染飞溅的血液或体液等时，应戴手套，条件允许时应戴口罩、眼罩及隔离衣。

（2）处理尖锐物品时要小心，切勿回套尖锐物。

（3）如果救护过程中使用了锐利性物品，使用后应进行妥善处理，防止发生针刺伤。

（4）救护人员在实施救治后，应进行手卫生，如戴手套，则应该脱掉手套后进行手卫生，戴手套不能代替洗手。

三、手卫生相关知识

如手部未见明显污染，可使用速干手消毒液进行手卫生；如手部有明显污染应使用流动水洗手。

（一）用速干手消毒液消毒双手步骤

1. 取足量（≥3ml）的速干手消毒液于掌心。

2. 涂抹双手，确保完全覆盖所有皮肤。

3. 按照六步洗手法揉搓，增加手腕部揉搓，时间至少20秒，揉搓至彻底干燥。

（二）流动水洗手步骤

1. 流动水下充分湿手。

2. 取洗手液（或肥皂）涂抹双手，完全覆盖所有皮肤。

3. 按照七步洗手法揉搓，双手揉搓时间不少于15秒。

4. 冲洗。

5. 干燥。

洗手全程时间应为40～60秒。

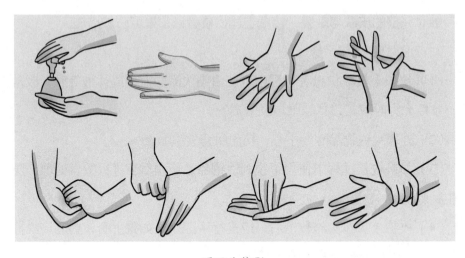

手卫生指引

四、不同传播途径感染性疾病的防护措施

1. 空气传播

空气传播是指病原体从传染源排出后，通过空气侵入新的易感宿主所经

历的全部过程。经空气传播的疾病包括肺结核、麻疹、水痘等。急救人员在处理该类患者时需佩戴医用防护口罩，并按规范脱防护口罩，做好手卫生。

飞沫传播是空气传播的一种，是指感染者在呼吸、咳嗽、打喷嚏时将带有病原体的口鼻腔飞沫喷射出来被易感者吸入，从而引起疾病传播的方式。是呼吸道传染病的主要传播途径。

可通过飞沫传播的疾病如流行性感冒、百日咳、严重急性呼吸综合征（SARS）等。急救人员需佩戴外科口罩，穿隔离衣（条件允许时），做好手卫生。

2. 接触传播

接触传播是指病原体通过媒介物直接或间接接触造成的传播。

可通过接触传播的疾病如肠道感染（腹泻）、多重耐药菌感染、皮肤感染（脓疱病）等。急救人员需佩戴手套，穿隔离衣（条件允许时），做好手卫生。

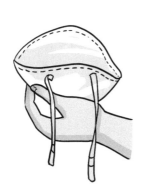
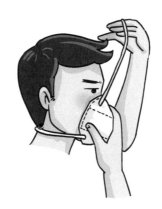

正确佩戴医用防护口罩

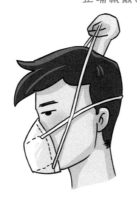
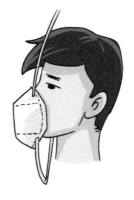

正确脱医用防护口罩

五、血液/体液暴露后的紧急处理

急救时，如发生血液/体液暴露需进行紧急处理，不同类型的暴露需采取不同的处理原则。

1. 针刺伤

流动水下冲洗约5分钟后，用碘伏等消毒剂消毒处理。

2. 皮肤破损、黏膜损伤

立即用大量流动水或生理盐水反复冲洗至少10分钟。

以上事件后均需立即报告医院感染控制部门进行处理。

六、污染物品和废物的处理及处置

完成施救程序后，所有用后可丢弃的急救物品及废弃物必须丢弃至指定的塑料袋内，打包封口，条件允许时可移交给专业人员，按照生活垃圾及医疗废物两大类进行分类和处置。

Chapter 1

Overview of Emergency Rescue

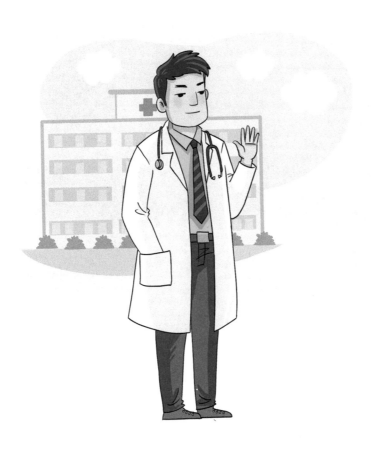

Definition

First aid, namely emergency rescue, refers to the provision of preliminary, timely, and effective rescue measures for the sick and the wounded at the scene of sudden accidents or disasters, before professional personnel arrive.

Characteristics

On-site, primary, mass-based emergency rescue.

Objectives

1. Save Lives

Take any first aid measures to save the lives of the sick and the wounded.

2. Prevent Deterioration

Prevent further development of injuries and secondary injuries to reduce disabilities.

3. Promote Recovery

Promote the physical and psychological recovery of the sick and the wounded.

First Aid Principles

1. Ensure Safety

Exclude hazardous factors, ensure environmental safety; take self-protection measures, wear protective gloves and protective clothing when necessary.

2. Prevent Infection

Avoid direct contact with secretions, blood, and body fluids of the sick and the wounded.

3. Take Reasonable Rescue

Save lives before treating injuries. Quickly determine whether there are head, chest, or abdominal fatal injuries. Keep the airway open. Apply pressure to stop bleeding before bandaging.

Proper Call for Assistance

When carrying out emergency first aid in a race against time, dial the emergency number "120" as soon as possible or seek help from surrounding bystanders.

Information to Report on the Phone:

(1) The specific location of the sick and the wounded, the obvious landmarks and buildings around, etc.

(2) The age, gender, and number of the sick and the wounded.

(3) The basic conditions of the sick and the wounded, such as massive bleeding, coma, chest pain, vomiting, dyspnea, etc.

(4) Possible causes of accident, such as traffic accidents, drowning, electric shock, poisoning, etc.

(5) Name and telephone number of the reporter.

(6) Ask for the approximate arrival time of the ambulance and be ready for pickup.

Answer the questions of the phone operator clearly and accurately, and wait for the operator to indicate that the call can be ended before hanging up.

Chapter 2

Legal Knowledge Related to First Aid

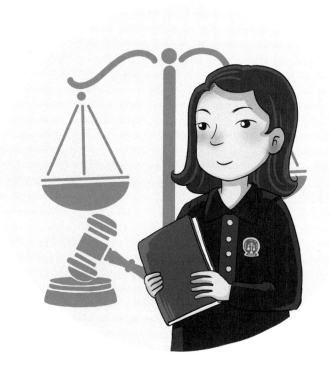

The legal safeguards and risks of first aid introduced in this chapter refer only to social first aid, that is, the activities of rescuing patients performed by non-medical emergency personnel on the spot.

Helping others in need is the fine tradition of the Chinese nation. Unfortunately, in recent years, incidents involving good Samaritans getting hurt or embroiled in legal disputes have caused the public to be wary of providing assistance.

The Article 184 in *General Provisions of the Civil Law of the People's Republic of China* (which implemented on October 1, 2017), commonly known as "Good Samaritan Law", states that a person who voluntarily provides emergency assistance and causes harm to the recipient of assistance shall not assume civil liability (After the *General Provisions of the Civil Law* were repealed, this provision was reflected in Article 184 of the *Civil Code of the People's Republic of China*). The *Regulations of Shenzhen Special Economic Zone on Emergency Medical Aid* was implemented on October 1, 2018, the Article 51 states that prior to the arrival of the emergency medical staff, any person on the scene with first aid capabilities is encouraged to provide first aid. This demonstrates the government's clear encouragement of such actions.

However, encouragement alone is not enough. Ordinary people, who are not legally obligated to provide assistance, may still face the following problems:

1. What if I provide aid, but the person is not saved, or I cause secondary injuries during the rescue?

According to the *Regulations on the Protection of the Rights and Interests of Rescuers in Shenzhen Special Economic Zone*, implemented on August 1, 2013, Article 4 states that the person being rescued must provide evidence to prove that the rescuer did not exercise reasonable care during the rescue process and caused further damage. If there is no evidence or insufficient evidence, the person being rescued shall bear the unfavorable consequences. Thus, if the rescuer has fulfilled his/her reasonable duty of care during the rescue, he/she will not be held legally responsible even if he/she has caused damage.

2. What if I provide aid and am falsely accused?

According to Article 3 of the *Regulations on the Protection of the Rights and Interests of Rescuers in Shenzhen Special Economic Zone*, the person being rescued must provide evidence to prove that his/her injury was caused by the rescuer. If there is no evidence or insufficient evidence, the person being rescued shall bear the unfavorable consequences. Article 5 states that if a rescuer incurs expenses due to false accusations by the person being rescued, the rescuer has the right to seek compensation according to the law. Article 6 stipulates that if the person being rescued falsely accuses the rescuer and violates public security regulations, he/she will be subject to administrative penalties; if his/her actions constitute a crime, he/she will be held criminally responsible. The rescuer can file a civil lawsuit against the person being rescued, who will then be held civilly responsible for making an apology, compensation for loss, elimination of adverse effects and rehabilitation of reputation.

3. What if I get injured while providing aid?

Implemented on January 1, 2013, the *Guangdong Province Regulations on Rewarding and Protecting Good Samaritans* provides comprehensive protection for those recognized as good Samaritans, including spiritual, honorary, and economic support, such as medical expenses.

In summary, to eliminate rescuers' concerns, the law protects those who provide well-intentioned, voluntary, and reasonable emergency assistance and exempts them from liability.

However, it is essential to emphasize that ordinary citizens without legal obligations to provide aid should always carry out rescue under the premise of ensuring their own safety. If the situation is assessed to be risky or if the individual is incapable of providing assistance, it is recommended to call "110" to report the incident or "120" to notify professional emergency personnel.

Chapter 3

CPR and AED

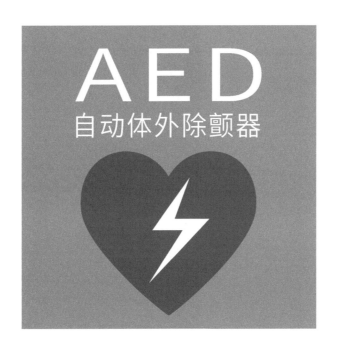

Sudden cardiac arrest has become a serious public health problem and one of the main causes of death in many regions of the world. It can occur both in and out of hospitals. This chapter focuses on the basic knowledge and skills required for non-medical personnel to perform cardiopulmonary resuscitation(CPR) outside the hospital, in order to improve the success rate of life-saving efforts in critical situations. The basic life support procedure is C-A-B (Chest compressions, Airway, Breathing).

Section 1   Adult CPR

Adult CPR Steps

1. Assessment

(1) Ensure the scene is safe for you and the patient.

(2) Gently tap the patient's shoulder and loudly ask, "Are you okay?"

(3) Check the patient's consciousness.

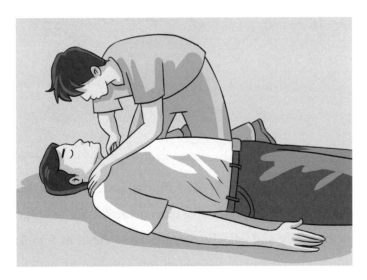

Assess the patient

2. Activate the Emergency Response System and Obtain an AED

(1) Seek help from others and dial the emergency phone number.

(2) Send someone to fetch or obtain an AED.

3. Assess Breathing

Observe the chest movement for 5 to 10 seconds, if there is no movement, sudden cardiac arrest can be assessed.

4. Initiate CPR

The rescuer should use compression-ventilation ratio of "30 : 2".

Chest compression skills:

(1) Kneel or stand on the patient's side with your legs apart.

(2) Ensure that the patient lies supine on a firm, flat surface, with the head, neck, and torso in a straight line.

(3) Place the heel of one hand on the center of the patient's chest.

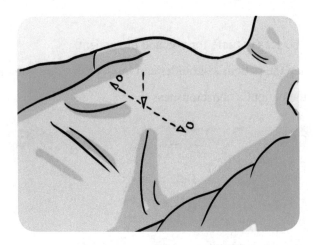

Chest compression location

(4) Place the heel of the other hand on the first hand and cross them firmly.

(5) Straighten both arms, positioning them perpendicular to the ground.

(6) Press forcefully and quickly, compress to a depth of 5 to 6 cm at a rate of 100 to 120 times per minute, ensuring full rebound of the chest wall and minimizing interruptions.

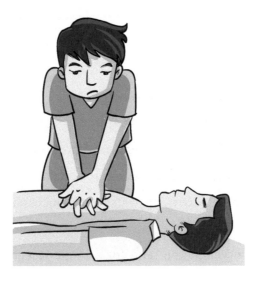

Chest compression position

(7) Open the airway for artificial respiration. Clear and open the airway. Use the head tilt-chin lift or jaw thrust method to open the airway. Perform mouth-to-mouth resuscitation or mouth-to-mask ventilation (or use a bag-valve-mask). Each artificial ventilation should raise the chest and be confirmed as effective ventilation.

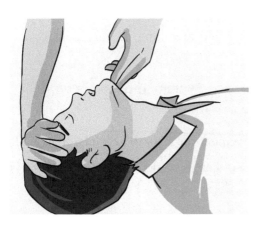

Head tilt-chin lift

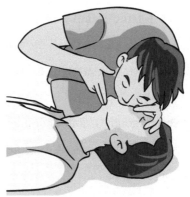

Mouth to mouth resuscitation

Section 2　Children and Infants CPR

Children CPR Steps

1. Assess the Scene Environment

2. Activate the Emergency Response System and Obtain AED

3. Assess the Child's Breathing and Reaction

Observe the chest and abdomen for 5 to 10 seconds. If no definite movement (that is no breathing) are felt, start CPR with chest compressions (C-A-B sequence).

4. Initiate CPR

The compression-ventilation ratio for a single rescuer is 30 : 2. For two rescuers, use a ratio of 15 : 2. Compress to a depth of about 5 cm, at a rate of 100 to 120 times per minute, ensuring full rebound of the chest wall and minimizing interruptions. Finally, open the airway and carry out two more times of artificial ventilations.

Infants CPR Steps

1. Assess the Scene Environment

Check for the infant's responsiveness and breathing. If unresponsive, no breathing, or only gasping, call for help.

2. Activate the Emergency Response System and Obtain an AED

3. Assess the Infant's Breathing

Observe the chest and abdomen movement for 5 to 10 seconds. Start CPR with chest compressions (C-A-B sequence) if there is no definite movement (that is no breathing).

4. Initiate CPR

(1) One-handed chest compression: Use a compression-ventilation ratio of 30 : 2 by placing two fingers on the center of the infant's chest, just below the nipple line, without pressing the lower end of the sternum.

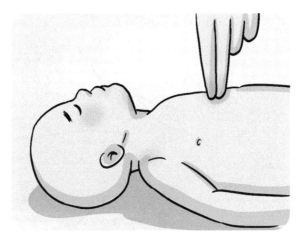

One-handed chest compression

(2) Two-thumb encircling technique: Place both thumbs side by side on the lower half of the infant's sternum on the center of the chest, with hands encircling the infant's chest, and use the other fingers to support the infant's back. The compression-ventilation ratio is 15∶2.

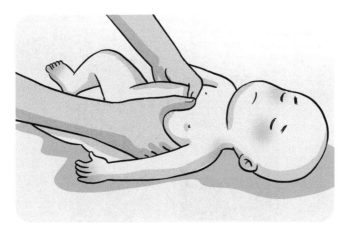

Two-thumb encircling technique

For each compression, press to a depth of about 4 cm (about 1/3 of the anterior-posterior diameter of the chest wall) at a rate of 100 to 120 times per minute, ensuring full rebound of the chest wall and minimizing interruptions.

5. Open the Airway and Perform Artificial Ventilation

Use the head tilt-chin lift technique to open the airway and provide mouth-to-mouth resuscitation or mouth-to-mask ventilation.

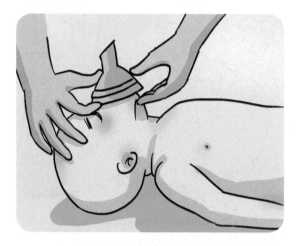

Mouth-to-mask ventilation

Section 3   AED Operation

AED Operation Steps

(1) Turn on the AED.

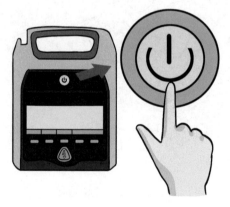

Turn on the power

(2) Apply the age-appropriate and right-size electrode pads to the patient according to the diagram, and connect the lead wires.

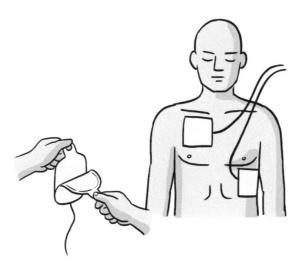

Stick the electrode pads

(3) Dismiss people around the patient and use the AED to analyse the patient's heart rhythm.

(4) Follow the AED's prompts, if electric shock is needed, press the "Charge " button. After the charging is complete and everyone has left, press the "Discharge" button, then start CPR immediately. If the AED indicates "No Shock Needed", continue CPR.

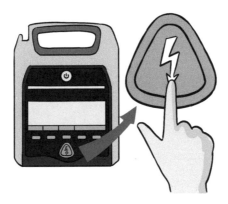

Electric shock

(5) Do not turn off the AED during CPR.

(6) Ensure the safety of rescuers when administering an electric shock.

(7) If performing two-person CPR, rescuers should switch roles during the AED analysis phase.

Chapter 4

On-the-Spot Trauma Rescue

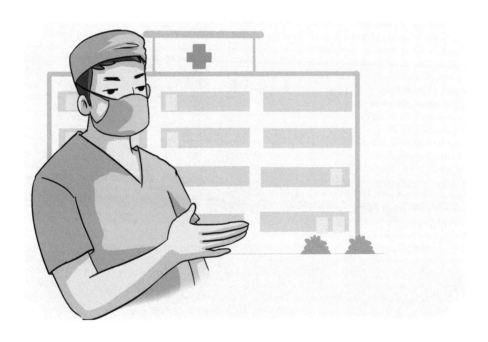

Trauma mainly refers to the injuries caused by mechanical force acting on the human body. Trauma is a medical subject that is both ancient and young. It is ancient because it has existed since the birth of mankind. It is young because with social progress and medical development, trauma continues to increase rather than decrease and is referred to as the "twin brother " of modern civilization.

Trauma can be classified as open or closed trauma based on whether the integrity of the body surface structure is destroyed. The degree of injury can be reduced as much as possible with proper on-site treatment of open trauma. The following first aid measures can assist you in effectively treating open trauma.

Section 1   Bleeding Treatment of Open Trauma

Open trauma includes skin damage, ruptures of blood vessels and nerve, fractures, etc., bleeding is very common, among which external bleeding is visible to the naked eye, as long as it's not the large artery bleeding, the injured often has a greater chance of being saved. The most common method used to stop bleeding from trauma is compression bandage method, which can be applied to wounds on the head, limbs, and other parts of the body. This method can be applied right away if immediate medical attention is not available.

Correct Methods of Hemostasis

1. Direct Wound Compression

Use a sufficiently thick, large and clean dressing to continuously cover the wound. The dressing should extend 3 to 4 cm beyond the wound.

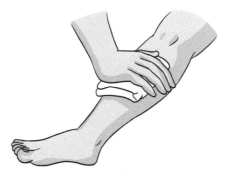

Compression hemostasis

2. Digital Pressure Hemostasis

Press your fingers on the bone near the proximal end of the bleeding artery (closer to the heart) to block the source of blood flow and achieve hemostasis.

(1) Bleeding from the top of the head and temporal region: On the injured side in front of the ear, use the index finger or thumb to press on the same side superficial temporal artery pulsation point.

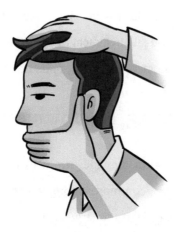

Superfacial temporal artery compression

(2) Facial bleeding: For bleeding on one side of the face, use the index finger or thumb to press on the same side facial artery pulsation point. The facial artery is about 3 cm in front of the angle of mandible, below the lower edge of the mandible.

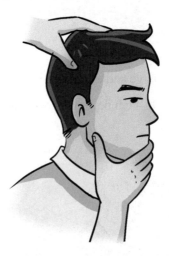

Facial artery compression

(3) Upper limb bleeding: Compress the axillary artery (armpit area) or the brachial artery against the humerus, and elevate the affected limb.

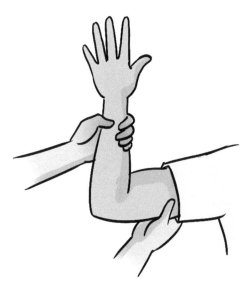

Brachial artery compression

(4) Palm bleeding: Compress the radial and ulnar arteries in the wrist.

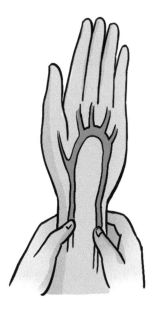

Radial and ulnar arteries compression

(5) Finger bleeding: Use the thumb and index finger to simultaneously compress the arteries on both sides.

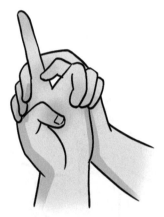

Digital artery compression

Bandaging

Utilize all available sterilized or clean, soft materials, such as towel, soft cloth, and clothing, etc., to achieve timely bandaging. The principle of bandaging is to cover first, then wrap, with moderate pressure. First, place a dressing (such as a sufficiently large and thick cotton pad) or gauze over the wound, and then use a bandage or triangular bandage to wrap it. The pressure should be moderate to ensure effective hemostasis and the distal artery is still pulsating; if the bandage is too loose, it will not stop the bleeding; if it is too tight, it can cause ischemia, hypoxia, or necrosis in the distal tissue.

1. Pressure Dressing

For body surface and limb injuries with bleeding, most can be temporarily stopped through pressure dressing and elevation of the limb. Apply sterile dressings or padding over the wound, and use hands or other objects to exert pressure on the dressings; the most common methods include padding with a bent elbow or bent knee, which usually taking 5 to 15 minutes to be effective. At the same time, elevating the injured area aids in stopping the bleeding; this method is suitable for small arteries, medium and small veins, or capillary bleeding.

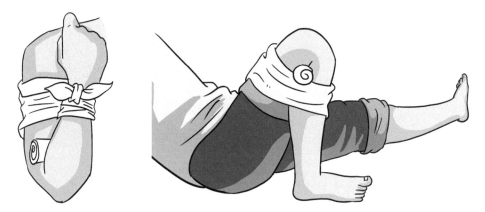

Padded bent-elbow hemostasis　　　Padded bent-knee hemostasis

If foreign bodies are found in the wound, follow these principles: ① shallow objects can be removed; ② deep objects should not be extracted (not removed), instead, fix the foreign body and bandage it.

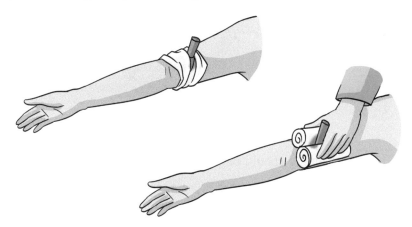

Deep foreign bodies bandaging

If there is spurting blood from the limb wound, it is necessary to use tourniquets to stop bleeding, which can be replaced with cloth tapes, ropes, triangular bandages, or towels, known as the tourniquet method. A small stick can also be added to tighten the knot, known as the tape tightening hemostasis method.

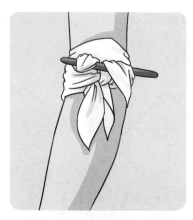

Tape tightening hemostasis

Moreover, a waist belt can be used to tighten and stop the bleeding.

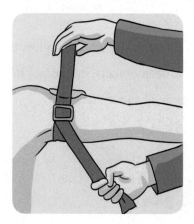

Hemostasis with a tightened belt

Note points: Padding should be under the tape; after tightening to stop the bleeding, record the time and relax once every 40 minutes. Plastic ropes, wires, and iron wires should not be used.

2. Bandage Wrapping

(1) Circular bandaging: This method is suitable for bandaging limbs of equal thickness and areas such as the chest and abdomen.

Specific method: Wrap the bandage in overlapping circles; the first circle should be slightly angled, and the second and third circles should be circular, pressing the angled corner of the first circle within the circular loops for more secure. Lastly, use adhesive tape to fix the tail end, or cut the tail into two and tie a knot.

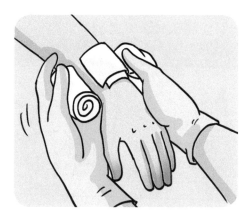

Circular bandaging

(2) Spiral bandaging: This method is suitable for bandaging limbs of unequal thickness.

Specific method: Begin by wrapping a few circles using the circular bandaging method to fix, then wrap upward, covering 1/3 or 2/3 of the front circle, forming a spiral shape. After completely covering the wound, wrap two more circles in place and fix.

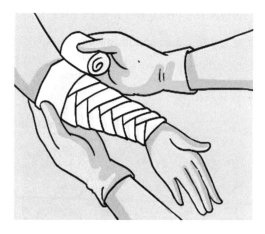

Spiral bandaging

(3) Figure 8 bandaging: Wrap the bandage above and below the joint in alternating circles, forming a figure 8 shape. Each circle intersects with the front one at the bend, and according to the situation, overlaps or covers 2/3 of the front circle.

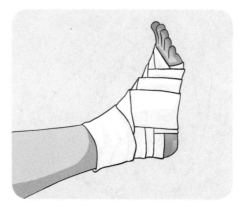

Figure 8 bandaging

(4) Open abdominal wounds bandaging: If there is an abdominal injury with exposed organs (such as intestines), follow these bandaging steps: ① The injured should be placed in supine position with both legs bent to relax the abdominal muscles as much as possible to prevent further organs prolapse; ② Cover the exposed organs with clean plastic or dressings, fix with adhesive tape around the edges, or place a clean bowl over them, then proceed with bandaging; ③ It is strictly prohibited to retract the prolapsed organs back into the abdominal cavity during the first aid, so as not to cause abdominal infection.

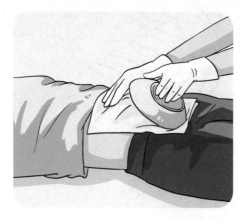

Bandaging of abdominal trauma with exposed organs

Note points: ① Stop the bleeding with pressure dressing on the wound. Cuts or scratches should be disinfected with povidone iodine and then covered with a

Band-Aid. ②Do not sprinkle any anti-inflammatory powders and other powders into the wound, and do not imprudently pull out the objects that have penetrated the wound.

Section 2   Treatment of Post-Traumatic Fractures

1. Limb Fractures

After a fracture occurs, fixation is a fundamental task in trauma care. Proper and effective fixation can quickly alleviate the patient's pain and reduce bleeding. At the scene, any available material can be utilized, such as splint, magazine, cardboard, wooden board, shoulder pole, stick, branch, bamboo, iron bar, or even belt and coat to fix the fractured part. If the aforementioned fixed materials are unavailable, the fractured limb can be fixed to the patient's trunk or healthy limb, using the trunk or healthy limb as a temporary splint. Common fracture treatments include the fixation of forearm and hand fractures, upper arm fractures, thigh fractures, and lower leg fractures.

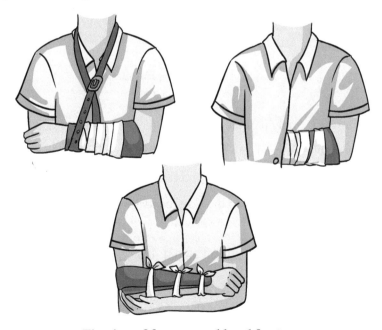

Fixation of forearm and hand fractures

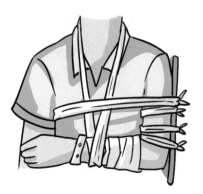

Fixation of upper arm fractures

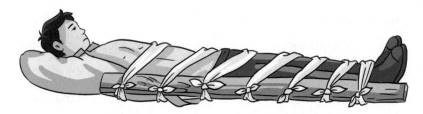

Fixation of thigh fractures

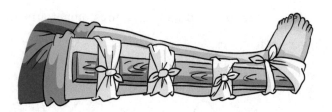

Fixation of lower leg fractures

Note points: ①Apply pressure dressing to the limb wound to stop bleeding, and look for any available material on-site to fix the fractured limb. When fixing, ensure that it extends beyond two joints above and below the injured limb. ②Do not push the exposed fractured end back into the skin, bandage it in situ and then fix it.

2. Spinal Fractures

After a traumatic injury, localized spinal pain, activity limitation, deformity, tenderness, and even incomplete or complete paralysis (such as the loss of sensation and motor function, or dysfunction of the urination and defecation) may indicate spinal injury, treatment should be more cautious. On the premise of environmental safety, remember not to move the patient imprudently, but always maintain the patient's spine in alignment.

Fixation for suspected cervical vertebrae fractures: Place two rolled-up towels on either side of the neck and tie them together. Ensure the tightness is appropriate and does not impede breathing.

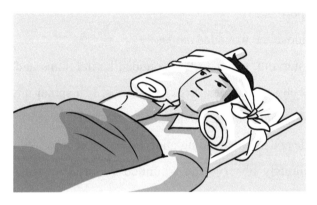

Fixation of suspected cervical vertebrae fractures

3. Pelvic Fractures

Pelvic fractures are severe traumas, more than half of which are accompanied by complications or multiple injuries, with a high rate of disability. Improper treatment can lead to a high mortality rate. Early external fixation is crucial for the rescue of hemorrhagic shock caused by pelvic fractures.

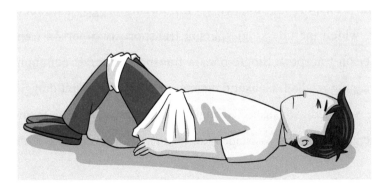

Fixation of pelvic fractures

Section 3　Transport of the Wounded

1. Principles for Transporting the Wounded

(1) First, assess whether the environment is safe, if not, move the wounded away from danger (emergency transport).

(2) When the environment is safe, stop bleeding, bandage and fix the wounded part before transport.

(3) Do not move the wounded aimlessly.

(4) Before moving, evaluate the wounded's vital signs and quickly inspect their head, neck, chest, abdomen, back, and limbs. If a spinal injury is suspected, fix the spine in alignment before moving.

(5) Be gentle and swift, avoiding unnecessary vibrations.

(6) Continuously observe the wounded's consciousness, breathing, and bleeding during transport.

(7) Explain to the wounded the method and purpose of the transport and obtain his/her cooperation.

2. Transport Methods

Transport can be classified as emergency transport and non-emergency transport. If the accident scene presents potential dangers or an unsafe environment, it is not advisable to administer first aid on the spot, but to carry the wounded to a safer and more comfortable place, and wait for medical assistance.

Manual transport methods rely on human strength without the use of equipment, which include single-person transport, two-person transport, and multiple-person transport. Single-person transport methods commonly involve clothing dragging method, blanket dragging method, and armpit dragging method, etc. For the wounded with suspected spinal injuries, avoid moving them rashly, but call for emergency medical assistance (unless there is a compelling reason to move them).

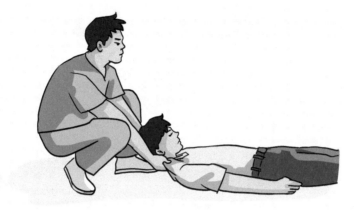

Clothing dragging method

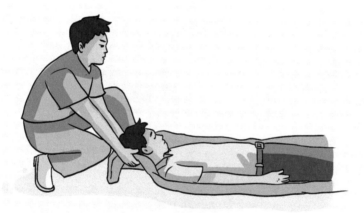

Blanket dragging method

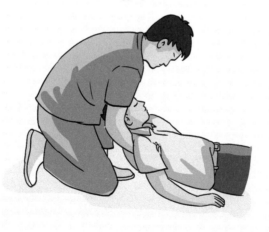

Armpit dragging method

Single-person transport methods

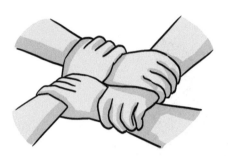

Two-person transport method

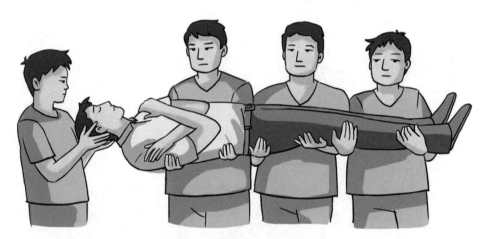

Multiple-person transport method

Chapter 5

First-Aid for Common Accidental Injuries

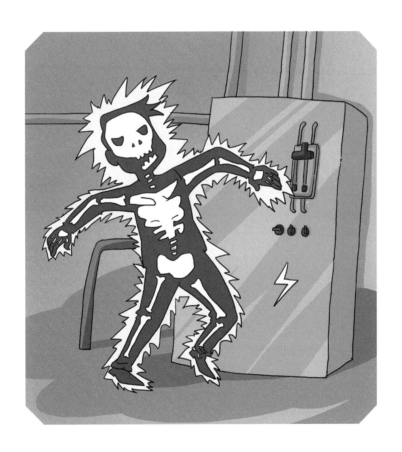

Section 1　Burns and Scalds

Overview

Burns and scalds refer to tissue injuries caused by direct or indirect heat (such as chemicals, electricity, radiation, etc.) acting on the body. They mainly refer to skin and mucosal injuries, and in severe cases can also damage the skin and submucosal tissue structures, such as muscles, bones, joints and even viscera.

Symptoms

Burn depth can be classified into four categories： I degree, superficial II degree, deep II degree and III degree according to the rule of three degrees and four levels.

I degree burn: Mainly damage the stratum corneum of the skin, causing local mild redness and swelling, no blisters, obvious pain.

Superficial II degree burn: Can reach the dermis, with blisters and severe pain.

Deep II degree burn: Small blisters with high density, skin ulceration.

III degree burn: Dry skin, local waxy white, brown or charcoal black, pain disappears.

Small-area superficial burns may cause local redness, swelling, heat, and pain of the burn, but the whole body may have no changes. Generally, they can heal within a few days if not infected. Large-area deep burns can destroy the stability of the human body's internal environment, causing dysfunction in various systems, such as shock, abnormal liver and kidney function, local and systemic infections, septicemia, multiple organ dysfunction and failure, and even death.

First Aid Measures

Burn first aid measures can be summarized as "1 rinse, 2 remove, 3 soak, 4 cover, 5 send", do not apply medication.

Step 1: Rinse

Rinse with cold water or soak the scalded limb in clean, cold water for 15 to 30 minutes until there is no pain or burning sensation.

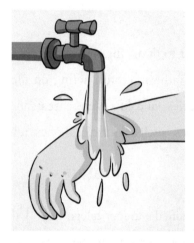

Rinse

Step 2: Remove

If the burn occurred while wearing close-fitting clothing, remove it after rinsing with cold water or use scissors to cut it open, and remove the clothing carefully. Do not forcibly peel off the clothing to avoid rupturing the blister. Remove any jewelry near the burn.

Step 3: Soak

For those with obvious pain, the scalded limb can be continuously immersed in cold water for 10 to 30 minutes, the main purpose is to relieve pain.

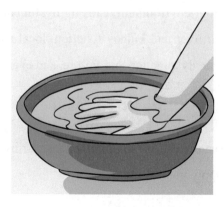

Soak

Step 4: Cover

Use a clean, sterile gauze or cotton cloth to cover the wound and fix it. This will help keep the wound clean and reduce external contamination.

Step 5: Send

Send the wounded to hospital for further treatment as soon as possible.

Section 2   Drowning

Overview

(1) Drowning is a common cause of death due to accidental injury, especially among adolescents.

(2) Asphyxia and hypoxia are the main causes of drowning-related death.

(3) Rescuers should ensure their own safety first, and then attempt to rescue the victim in the water. Entering the water to rescue the victim may lead to drowning oneself.

(4) Priority should be given to open the airway and artificial respiration in drowning first aid.

Drowning Chain of Survival

(1) Prevent drowning: Be safe in and around water.

(2) Recognize distress: Ask someone to call for help.

(3) Provide flotation: To prevent submersion.

(4) Remove from water: Only if safe to do so.

(5) Provide care as needed: Seek medical attention.

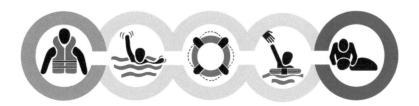

Drowning chain of survival

Rescue Measures In Water

Prevent Drowning	*Be safe in and around the water* 1. Stay within arm's reach of children when in or near the water 2. Swim where there are lifeguards 3. Always wear a lifejacket when using watercraft 4. Learn how to swim and water-safety survival skills	
Recognize Distress	*Ask someone to call for help* 1. Recognise early drowning victim's distress signs (Victims may not wave or call for help) 2. Tell someone to call for help while staying on-scene to provide assistance	
Provide Flotation	*To prevent submersion* While helping others: 1. Stay out of the water to reduce rescuer risk 2. Throw something that floats to the victim To help yourself: 1. If you are in difficulty, don't panic; stay with any flotation you may have 2. Signal for help as soon as and if possible, and float	
Remove from Water	*Only if safe to do so* 1. Assist the victim on how to self-rescue by giving them directions for getting out of the water 2. Try to remove the victim without entering the water	
Provide Care as Needed	*Seek medical attention* 1. If not breathing, start CPR (ventilations and compressions) immediately 2. Consider the use of oxygen and an AED as soon as possible if available 3. If breathing, stay with victim until help arrives 4. Seek medical aid/hospital if any symptoms are present, and for all victims who require resuscitation	

Rescue Measures Out of Water

Safety	Consider your own safety first, avoid entering the water.
Pacify the victim	*Talk to the victim, encourage him/her to rescue himself/herself:* 1. Do not be flustered, be sure to keep your head clear. 2. Take the top of the head backwards, the mouth upwards, and expose the nose and mouth to the surface of the water. At this time, you can breathe. 3. Exhale should be shallow, and the inhalation should be deep, so that the body floats on the water as much as possible to wait for rescue. 4. Do not lift or struggle with your hands, which is easy to sink people.
Reach the victim	Build a bridge with the drowning person by means of branches, sticks, ropes or clothing.
Throw floating objects	Throw floating objects to the drowning person, which can be wood, lifebuoy, ball, empty water bottle with lid.
Use boat	If you can use a boat, consider boat rescue.
Self-help	*If you can swim:* (1) The swimmer may be drowning due to calf gastrocnemius muscle spasm, you should be calm, and promptly call for help. (2) Pull yourself together and float to the surface. (3) Take a deep breath, immerse your face in the water, pull the toe of the spasmodic lower forward and upward, so that the thumb is warped up and continue to sustained exertion until the pain is gone, and the cramping stop. (4) After an episode, the same part can be cramped again, so massage the pain area and slowly swim to the shore. After landing, it's best to massage and warm compress the affected area. (5) If the wrist muscles cramp, you can bend your fingers up and down, and take the back position with two feet swimming. *If you cannot swim:* If unable to swim, the drowning person should swims back to the shore with life-saving appliances (lifebuoy, etc.)
Others-help	The rescuer should approach from behind, hold the head and neck of the drowning person from behind with one hand, and the other hand grabs the arm of the drowning person and swims to the shore.

Section 3   Electric Shock Injuries

Electric shock injuries, commonly known as electrocution, occur when a certain amount of electric current or electric energy (static electricity) passes through the human body, causing varying degrees of tissue injuries or dysfunctions. Severe cases can result in sudden cardiac arrest or respiratory arrest.

What should you do if you find someone electrocuted?

(1) Confirm the safety of the environment at the scene.

(2) Help the victim quickly disconnect from the power source.

1) Turn off the power: pull out the power plug or pull down the power switch.

2) Remove the electrical wire: use insulating materials or dry wooden sticks, bamboo poles, or shoulder poles to remove the wire.

3) Pull the victim away: wear rubber shoes and stand on a wooden stool or plank, use a dry rope, scarf, or dry clothes twisted into a strip to pull the victim away. Do not touch the victim's body directly.

(3) Call out the victim and observe the chest movement for 5 to 10 seconds, if no breathing and reaction, start CPR immediately.

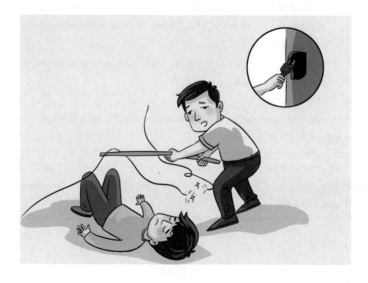

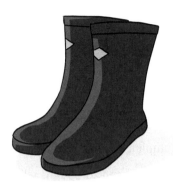
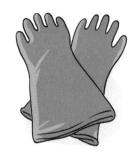

Insulating materials

(4) If the victim has extensive burns, protect the wound.

(5) Dial the emergency number "120" quickly.

Section 4   Epistaxis and Airway Foreign Body

Epistaxis

When epistaxis occurs, pinch both sides of the wing of nose for 10 to 15 minutes while applying a cold water pack or wet towel to the forehead or back of the neck to reduce bleeding. If the amount of bleeding is large, seek medical attention promptly.

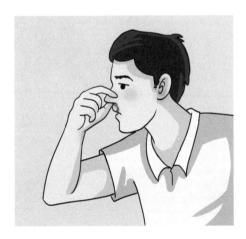

Epistaxis

Airway Foreign Body

1. Adult-Rescue

(1) Rescuing others: After getting stuck by an airway foreign body, it is necessary to first identify incomplete or complete foreign body airway obstruction. In the former case, the victim should be encouraged to cough, while in the latter case, the Heimlich maneuver should be applied immediately. If the victim is awake, the rescuer can stand with the "front leg bent, back leg straight" posture, allowing the person to lean forward slightly, and embrace the patient with both arms under the patient's armpits. One hand should make a fist, with the other hand grasping the first hand. Place the fist just above the navel in the center of the abdomen and then suddenly tighten both arms, applying strong pressure upward and inward, causing the abdomen to collapse. Repeat this action until the foreign body is discharged.

Put the victim in a supine position on the ground if he/she has lost consciousness, start CPR right away.

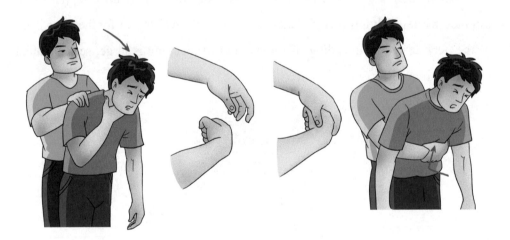

Gestures

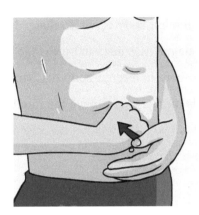

Heimlich maneuver

(2) Self-rescue: If there is no one around in an emergency situation, the self-rescue method can be used. The patient can make a fist with the left hand, grasp the left fist with the right hand from the front, place the left fist in the center of the abdomen just above the navel, and then exert force with both arms, or use a blunt object to apply quick upward pressure to the abdomen to expel the foreign body, such as by rapidly impacting the abdomen while leaning against the back of a chair.

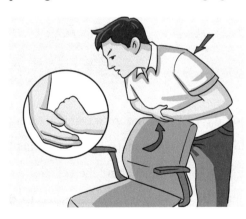

Self-rescue

2. Infant-Rescue

Gently pick up the infant, pinch both sides of the zygomatic bone with one hand, while the arm rests against the infant's chest. Support the back of the infant's neck with the other hand. Carefully place the infant face down and on the rescuer's lap. Pat the infant 5 times on the shoulder and back and observe whether the foreign body is discharged. If the foreign body is not discharged, turn over the infant, and put the index and middle fingers together, and press the lower end of the sternum 5 times. Observe whether there is foreign body discharge from the mouth at any time. If the foreign body is discharged, remove the foreign body with fingers. The above actions should be done with the infant's head below the chest. If that is not effective, the above actions can be repeated.

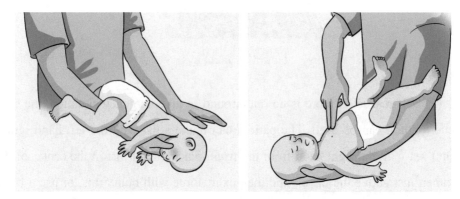

Infant-rescue

Section 5   Traffic Accident

Accident Handling at the Scene

(1) The driver should turn on the hazard warning flashers immediately.

(2) Move the vehicle to a location that does not obstruct traffic.

(3) Put a warning sign 150 meters behind the vehicle.

(4) The driver and the passengers should move to the right shoulder or emergency lane quickly.

(5) Call the emergency number "122" right away.

(6) Protect the scene and maintain order.

On-the-Spot Rescue

1. CPR

Assess the victim for 5 to 10 seconds. If there is no breathing, perform CPR directly.

2. Control Bleeding

(1) Direct pressure: Apply pressure directly to the wound with palm or fingers and maintain for more than 15 minutes.

(2) Elevation: Raise the injured limb so that the bleeding site is higher than the heart to slow the blood flow.

(3) Compression hemostasis: When there is severe bleeding in the limbs, apply pressure to the main arteries of the limbs.

3. Transport the Wounded

(1) Do not move the wounded rashly, especially when cervical or lumbar spine fractures.

(2) Hemostasis and fixation before handling, you can use hard branches on site, and perform bandaging and fixation with clothes before moving.

(3) Waiting for medical professionals to arrive for treatment.

Section 6　Poisoning

Overview

Poisoning refers to the toxic chemicals enter the human body through certain routes and interact with the body, directly causing changes in the function or structure of the body through biophysical or biochemical reactions, resulting in temporary or permanent damage, or even life-threatening diseases. Whether poisoning occurs after the poisons enter the body depends on various factors, such as the toxicity, properties, amount and time of entry of the poisons into the body, and individual differences (such as sensitivity and tolerance to the poisons) of the patient.

Emergency Treatment for Different Types of Poisoning

1. Cleansing Agent

Examples include dishwashing detergent, disinfectant, and kitchen cleaner, etc. The severity of poisoning is related to the amount ingested. Small amounts mainly cause gastrointestinal irritation, while large amounts can cause gastrointestinal corrosion, coma, convulsion, and other symptoms.

Treatment: Go to the hospital immediately, turn the patient's head to one side if unconscious, to prevent aspiration.

2. Desiccant

(1) Silica gel: translucent beads, insoluble in water. If accidentally ingested, no special treatment is needed, as they are generally considered non-toxic or low-toxic.

(2) Calcium oxide: A white or grayish-white powder that dissolves in water to form calcium hydroxide, which is highly corrosive.

(3) Calcium chloride: commonly used for moisture absorption in closets, plastic packaging, appears as white granules or flocculent. It dissolves in humid environments and is highly corrosive.

Treatment:

(1) If the toxicant is ingested within 30 minutes, water, milk and egg white, etc. can be given for dilution and protection.

(2) If the composition of the poison is unclear, bring the poison and seek medical attention as soon as possible.

3. Insect Repellent Pills

Common ingredients in insect repellent pills include camphor, naphthalene, and dichlorobenzene, among which camphor and naphthalene are highly toxic.

Treatment: Bring the poison and seek medical attention as soon as possible.

4. Alcoholism

Alcohol can be rapidly absorbed in the stomach and small intestine, and the concentration of alcohol can be detected in the blood 5 minutes after drinking. According to relevant statistics, the average lethal dose of alcohol for adults is 250 to 500 grams. The severity of alcohol poisoning is related to the amount ingested, generally causing gastrointestinal irritation, mild neural suppression symptoms, etc. In severe cases, it can cause coma and convulsion.

Treatment:

(1) Mainly prevent suffocation caused by vomiting, conscious patients can drink sugar water.

(2) If a large amount of alcohol has been consumed and the patient's reaction is significantly milder than usual, seek medical attention immediately.

Section 7   Animal-Induced Injuries

Overview

Different types of animals cause injuries to human body through different ways, and such injuries have high individual specificity.

Emergency Treatment for Different Types of Animal Bites

1. Mammal Bites

Bite marks or lacerated wounds with irregular edges. The severity depends on the size, location, and contamination of the wound.

Treatment:

(1) Clean the wound simply, and apply appropriate bandaging and fixation. Do not attempt to remove foreign bodies without confidence.

(2) Since the teeth of animals (such as cats and dogs) carry many bacteria and viruses, in addition to conventional wound treatment, it is best to go to a nearby hospital for treatment.

2. Snake Bites

Treatment:

(1) Calm the patient, keeping him/her composed, and avoiding panic or running.

(2) Immediately tie a soft rope or cloth strip around the injured limb, about 5 cm above the wound and closer to the heart. Loosen the tie for 1 to 2 minutes

every 15 to 30 minutes to avoid ischemic necrosis of tissue, and fix the affected limb.

(3) For venomous snake bites, after emergency treatment, the patient must be quickly sent to a regular hospital for further standardized emergency treatment.

Note points: All snakebite victims must be sent to the hospital as soon as possible.

3. Insect Stings/Bites

The main symptoms include local burning pain, swelling, redness, itch at the site of the injury, and some specific insects can even cause asthma attacks, dyspnea, or coma.

Treatment:

(1) After being stung, if toxic hairs or sting ends are found on the skin, remove them with tweezers.

(2) Rinse the site of sting with flowing cold water carefully and apply a cold compress.

(3) If the stung site has obvious redness and pain, take the victim to the nearest hospital as soon as possible.

Note points: Carefully observe for signs of anaphylactic shock.

4. Jellyfish Stings

Symptoms include redness, pain, itching at the stung site, accompanied by rash, and severe cases may present dyspnea, muscle spasm, or coma.

Treatment:

(1) Leave the water as soon as possible after being stung by jellyfish.

(2) Rinse the wound with seawater (do not use freshwater or touch the tentacles with your hand) and apply a cold compress to alleviate pain.

(3) Seek medical help immediately for severe stings.

Chapter 6

Common Emergency Rescue

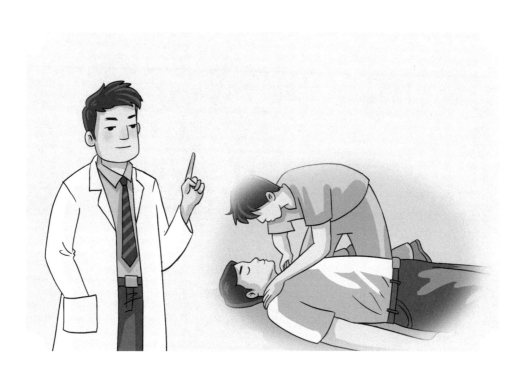

Section 1　Asthma

Overview

Asthma is a chronic inflammatory disease of the airway. Clinically, patients with asthma present with recurrent episodes of wheezing, coughing, chest distress, and tachypnea. Asthma attacks can happen at any time but are especially common at night and in the morning. Severe asthma attacks may be life-threatening and usually require immediate medical attention.

Key Points of First Aid

(1) Prepare medications and inhaler devices for the patient quickly, and help the patient apply fast-acting symptom-relief medications.

(2) Help the patient find the most comfortable position (which is usually sitting position), leaning slightly forward, and resting on his/her elbows or arms to breathe.

(3) Leave one person to comfort and accompany the patient, avoiding multiple people standing around the patient, so as not to make the patient more anxious.

(4) Call "120" (emergency number) immediately, calmly and quickly transport the patient to the nearest hospital.

Section 2　Chest Pain

Overview

Chest pain is a common and critical clinical symptom with various causes, and most of them are chest diseases. The common emergencies that cause chest pain are as follows.

1. Coronary Heart Disease (CHD)

Coronary heart disease is more likely to occur in people with "three highs" (hypertension, hyperglycemia, hyperlipidemia), long-term smoking, obesity, and those with a family history of CHD. Chest pain of CHD typically presents as pain behind the sternum, accompanied by sweating, lasting for more than 5 minutes, and characterized by a suffocating pain and difficult breathing, as if a large stone is pressed on the chest.

2. Aortic Dissection

Hypertension is the main risk factor for aortic dissection, and substandard blood pressure control is the inducement. The pain of aortic dissection is often as severe as a knife cut and unbearable. Some people describe it as "the most painful experience in their life". The pain lasts for a long time, cannot be relieved by rest, and may also be accompanied by back pain and abdominal pain.

3. Pulmonary Embolism

If there are risk factors such as liver and kidney dysfunction, recent major surgery, long-term bed rest, or taking steroid medications, be vigilant for the possibility of pulmonary embolism. In addition to chest pain, pulmonary embolism typically also presents with symptoms such as difficult breathing, coughing up blood, coughing with phlegm, and in severe cases, may lead to faint and shock.

Key Points of First Aid

Chest pain is a serious disease, and the following points should be considered when facing chest pain.

(1) Take chest pain seriously and avoid adopting a "bear with it" attitude, as it may delay treatment.

(2) Call "120" (emergency number) immediately; it is not recommended to walk or take a vehicle to the hospital.

(3) Have the patient rest quietly in a lying position while waiting for medical personnel.

(4) Measure blood pressure and heart rate with a domestic blood pressure monitor and keep a record.

(5) For high-risk individuals with CHD, it is advisable to have emergency medications such as Suxiao Jiuxin pills, nitroglycerin tablets and nitroglycerin spray readily available at home. Use them as soon as chest pain appears.

Section 3   Stroke

Overview

Stroke, commonly known as "apoplexy", is an acute cerebrovascular disease that includes hemorrhagic stroke (cerebral hemorrhage) and ischemic stroke (cerebral infarction), with high mortality and disability rates. According to data, there are about 2 million new stroke patients in China every year, and there is a tend towards younger. In China, more than 1.5 million people die from stroke each year. Stroke has become the leading cause of death in China, exceeding all cancers combined. Pre-hospital delay is the main reason for the high mortality and disability rates of stroke in China.

How to Identify a Stroke

For stroke patients, time is life. How to identify stroke symptoms as early as possible? The formula "Stroke 120" was proposed by the Stroke 120 Special Task Force of Chinese Stroke Association, which is suitable for Chinese population to identify strokes quickly. "1" represents one face, whether the patient's face shows symptoms such as crooked mouth, facial numbness, or salivation; "2" represents two arms, when both arms are raised flat, observe whether there are symptoms of weakness or numbness on one side; "0" represents listening, observe whether there are symptoms such as slurred speech, speech difficulty, or inability to speak. If any of the above sudden symptoms are observed, call "120" immediately.

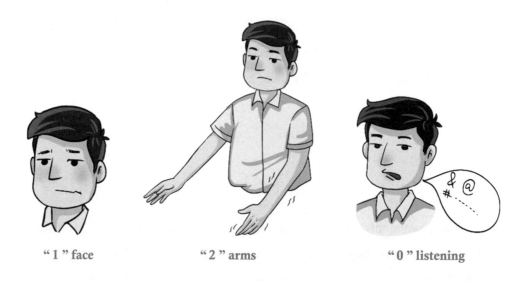

"1" face   "2" arms   "0" listening

What Will Doctors Do After the Patient Arrive at the Hospital

In general, doctors will immediately arrange the patient at the emergency room, connect to an electrocardiogram monitor, take blood tests, measure blood glucose, and perform a head CT scan as soon as possible.

If the head CT scan indicates no cerebral hemorrhage, the patient will be advised to undergo immediate pharmacological thrombolysis or even further interventional thrombectomy (may need to be transferred to a hospital with the necessary facilities); the use of thrombolytic drugs and interventional surgery requires the patient or family members to sign the relevant consent form.

If the head CT scan indicates cerebral hemorrhage, the doctor will decide on hospitalization or consultation with neurosurgeons, depending on the amount of bleeding, and proceed with surgery or interventional treatment.

During hospital treatment, maintaining stable vital signs is the foundation of treatment, so it may be necessary to perform tracheal intubation to maintain airway patency, perform deep vein puncture, use vasoactive drugs, provide ventilator-assisted ventilation, gastric intubation, and perform urethral catheterization.

How to Prevent Stroke

(1) Controlling blood pressure is the key to preventing stroke. Hypertensive patients should take antihypertensive medications on time, monitor blood pressure, maintain a light and moderate diet, quit smoking and limit alcohol consumption, exercise moderately, and maintain emotional stability.

(2) The key to the prevention and treatment of atherosclerosis is the prevention and treatment of hyperlipidemia and obesity.

(3) Control diabetes and other diseases such as heart disease, vasculitis and so on.

(4) Pay attention to the impact of meteorological factors: seasonal and climatic changes can cause emotional instability and blood pressure fluctuation in hypertensive patients, trigger strokes, and should be more vigilant against the occurrence of stroke at this time.

Section 4   Hypertension

Overview

Hypertension can be diagnosed in adults when their blood pressure exceeds 140/90mmHg three times in different days. The prevalence of hypertension in Chinese adults is as high as 25.2%, which means that 1 in 4 people have hypertension.

Dangers of Hypertension

Hypertension is a chronic disease and the most important risk factor of stroke, coronary heart disease and renal failure. According to statistics, 2 million people die from hypertension-related diseases in China each year, and more than 60% of coronary heart disease patients, more than 80% of cerebral infarction patients, and 90% of cerebral hemorrhage patients have a history of hypertension. It can be said that hypertension is an "invisible killer" of human health.

Symptoms of Hypertension

Hypertensive patients usually have no obvious symptoms. Common clinical symptoms include headache, dizziness, inattentiveness, memory loss, limb numbness, increased nocturia, palpitation, chest distress, and fatigue.

Common Problems about Hypertension

1. Is long-Term Use of Antihypertensive Drugs Addictive

Antihypertensive drugs are not addictive. Patients should take antihypertensive drugs regularly and reasonably under the guidance of a doctor, which will not cause damage to the body and will also help to control blood pressure.

2. Can Medication Be Stopped After Blood Pressure Is Controlled

Some hypertensive patients think that once antihypertensive drugs lower their blood pressure to normal, it means that hypertension has been cured and they can stop taking medicine. However, blood pressure may rise again after stopping medication, and intermittent medication can cause blood pressure fluctuation, which may lead to greater harm. Hypertensive patients should adjust the dosage and types of medication gradually and carefully under the guidance of a doctor, do not stop medication or change the dosage on their own.

3. Can Health Supplements Replace Antihypertensive Drugs

Some patients believe that Western medicine has significant side effects and are unwilling to take it long term. They rely on health supplements blindly because they have heard that some health supplements can lower blood pressure. In fact, the blood pressure-lowering effects of health supplements are not reliable. Although some health supplements have certain auxiliary blood pressure-lowering effects, they cannot replace antihypertensive drugs.

4. Can Dietary Therapy Alone Lower Blood Pressure

Diet is the foundation of hypertension treatment, and dietary interventions can delay the further rise of blood pressure, but it cannot achieve the goal of controlling blood pressure. Therefore, in most cases, blood pressure cannot be lowered by dietary therapy alone.

5. Can Patients Buy the Same Antihypertensive Drugs as Other Patients at the Pharmacy

Antihypertensive treatment plans vary between individuals, and patients should not follow other people's medication plans. Patients should monitor their blood pressure dynamically under the guidance of a doctor and adjust their medication according to their blood pressure levels.

6. What to Do if Blood Pressure Suddenly Rises

Under certain triggering factors, blood pressure may suddenly and significantly increase (generally above 180/120mmHg). If it is accompanied by progressive acute damage to important target organs such as heart, brain, or kidney, it is clinically called hypertensive emergencies; if there is no damage to target organs, it is called hypertensive urgencies.

Both situations are highly dangerous cardiovascular emergencies that require timely and effective treatment. Patients should go to the hospital immediately and receive specialist treatment to avoid serious complications.

Section 5   Shock

Overview

Shock is a syndrome caused by severe pathogenic factors attacking the body, leading to a sharp decrease in effective circulating blood volume, widespread, persistent, and significant reduction in tissue blood perfusion, poor microcirculation function, and severe dysfunction of vital organs.

Clinical Manifestations

The clinical manifestations of shock include decreased blood pressure, oliguria or even anuria, cold and clammy skin, mottled skin changes on limbs, and conscious disturbance.

Etiologies of Shock

The etiologies of shock include cardiogenic factors, allergic factors, infectious factors, and pulmonary embolism.

Shock is a common clinical emergency and life-threatening condition with a high mortality rate. Clinical manifestations appear late, and once hypotension occurs, the condition may have already worsened, necessitating immediate treatment. Effective intervention in the early stages of shock, controlling the primary causes of shock, and stopping the progression of the disease can help improve the patient's prognosis.

Section 6　Diabetes

Overview

Diabetes mellitus is a group of disorders of carbohydrate, protein, and fat metabolism caused by absolute and relative insulin deficiency, and/or insulin utilization disorders, with hyperglycemia as the main sign.

The human body can maintain a dynamic balance between the sources and destinations of blood glucose through two major regulatory systems: hormonal regulation and neural regulation, maintaining blood glucose at a certain level. However, under the combined action of genetic factors (such as a family history of diabetes) and environmental factors (such as an unreasonable diet and obesity), these two regulatory systems become disordered, resulting in an increase (hyperglycemic emergency) or decrease (hypoglycemic emergency) in blood glucose levels.

Clinical Manifestations

1. Manifestations of Hyperglycemic Emergency

Polydipsia, polyphagia, polyuria, weight loss, blurred vision, fatigue and drowsiness, etc.

2. Manifestations of Hypoglycemic Emergency

Hunger, dizziness, palpitation, hand shaking, cold sweat, sweating profusely, serious disturbance of consciousness, coma and even death.

3. Diabetic Complications

Such as retinopathy, stroke, acute myocardial infarction, atherosclerosis, peripheral neuropathy, diabetic nephropathy and so on.

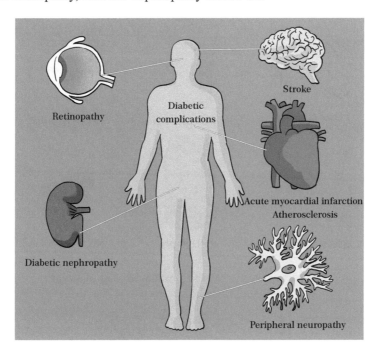

Emergency Treatment Measures

1. Treatment of Hyperglycemic Emergency

Patients who need insulin or other medications should be sent to the hospital immediately for blood glucose reduction treatment when experiencing the hyperglycemic emergency, and the blood glucose changes should be closely monitored. If the patient is unconscious, while being sent to the hospital, the patient should lie flat with his or her head turned to one side to prevent asphyxia.

2. Treatment of Hypoglycemic Emergency

(1) If the patient is conscious, help the patient sit or lie down; if the patient is unconscious, send him/her to the hospital immediately for treatment.

(2) When the patient can eat, give him/her fast-acting sugar-raising foods with 15g of sugar, and seek medical attention promptly when the patient's condition is stable. If the patient's condition does not improve, check the patient for other causes of coma, and send him/her to the hospital as soon as possible.

(3) Keep the patient's airway open, check the patient's breathing, pulse, and degree of responsiveness.

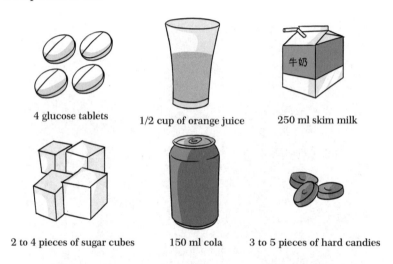

| 4 glucose tablets | 1/2 cup of orange juice | 250 ml skim milk |

| 2 to 4 pieces of sugar cubes | 150 ml cola | 3 to 5 pieces of hard candies |

Fast-acting sugar-raising foods with 15g of sugar

Section 7   Epilepsy

Overview

Epilepsy is a chronic disease caused by sudden abnormal discharge of brain neurons, which leads to transient brain dysfunction.

Emergency Treatment Measures

(1) Ensure the safety of the patient during an epileptic seizure. Move the patient away from high or dangerous places, making sure there are no sharp objects (including glasses) around the patient. If the patient has not yet fallen, immediately support him/her to maintain balance and gently help him/her lie down. The purpose

of this operation is to provide a safe space for the patient to prevent secondary injuries. Many clinical cases involve patients suffering from cerebral hemorrhage because of falling down during an epileptic seizure or being scalded when limbs spasm knocks over hot water.

(2) Ensure the patient's airway is clear. After the patient lies down, turn the patient to a lateral position or turn his/her head to one side if it's not convenient. This operation can effectively avoid aspiration of secretions into the airway by mistake and can also prevent the tongue from falling back and blocking the airway during a seizure. Aspiration of secretions or foreign bodies in the mouth and nose can cause asphyxia in a short time or lead to aspiration pneumonia later, so do not neglect this step.

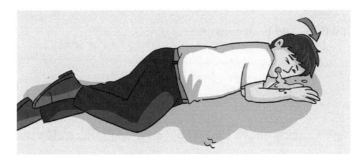

Lateral position

(3) If the patient wears a tie or clothes are too tight, loosen the tie and adjust or remove the tight clothing to facilitate breathing. Generally, epileptic seizures are self-limiting and will stop after a few minutes. However, common tonic-clonic seizure (the most common "grand mal") may last more than 5 minutes and enter a state of status epilepticus, requiring drug intervention to terminate the seizure.

Note points

(1) Pressing the "philtrum" cannot terminate an epileptic seizure.

(2) Do not put any object into the patient's mouth during a seizure to avoid asphyxia.

(3) Do not attempt to feed water before the patient regains consciousness, as this may cause aspiration.

(4) Do not forcefully press the patient's limbs during convulsions to avoid

fractures or sprains.

Section 8   Heatstroke

Overview

Heatstroke is an acute disease characterized by central nervous system and/or cardiovascular dysfunction due to dysfunction of the body temperature regulating center or sweat gland failure, as well as excessive loss of water and electrolytes in an airtight environment with high temperature or humidity. Symptoms may include dizziness, high fever (body temperature 39.1 to 41.0℃), reduced sweating, vomiting, palpitation, and limb convulsion.

Emergency Treatment Measures

Transfer: Quickly move the patient to a cool and well-ventilated area, elevate his/her head, and loosen his/her clothing.

Apply: Place cold towels or ice packs on his/her head, armpits, and the root of thighs.

Rub: Wipe the whole body with a cold towel.

Soak: For severe heatstroke patient, place him/her in cold water for immersion, while massaging his/her limbs to promote blood circulation and accelerate heat dissipation.

Section 9   Fever

Overview

Fever refers to the elevation of the body temperature due to the action of pyrogen, which raises the set-point of the body temperature regulating center. Fever degrees (take the oral temperature as the standard, axillary temperature is 0.3 to 0.5 ℃ lower than oral temperature) can be classified as low grade fever: 37.3 to 38.0℃ ; moderate fever: 38.1 to 39.0℃ ; high fever: 39.1 to 41.0℃ ; and extremely high fever: above 41.0℃ .

Clinical Manifestations

Fever can be divided into effervescence period, persistent febrile period and defervescence period, with different symptoms in different phases. During the effervescence period, patients usually experience fatigue and a certain degree of muscle soreness in the limbs or dry and pale skin, as heat production exceeds heat dissipation and body temperature continues to rise. During the persistent febrile period, the patient's body temperature remains at a higher level, accompanied by skin flushing, burning sensation, increased heart rate and respiration. The defervescence period is mainly characterized by profuse sweating and a decrease in skin temperature.

Emergency Treatment Measures

(1) If there are prodromal symptoms of febrile seizure, place a bite block between the upper and lower teeth to prevent biting the tongue.

(2) Loosen the patient's collar, turn the head to one side to facilitate the flow of secretions.

(3) Call "120" promptly.

Chapter 7

Disaster Escape and Rescue

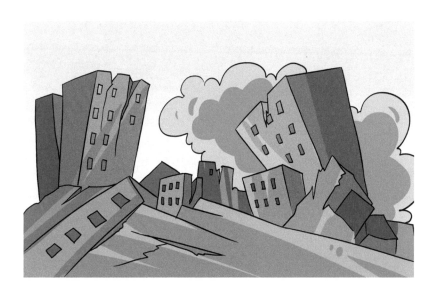

Natural disasters are sudden and often difficult to predict and prevent, therefore, causing extensive damage. Before a disaster occurs, we should master the knowledge of disaster prevention, learn basic self-rescue and mutual-rescue skills, and be mentally prepared. Once a disaster occurs, knowing how to escape and provide first aid can help reduce the losses caused by the disaster. This chapter focuses on the escape and first aid knowledge for several common disasters.

Section 1   Earthquake

Overview

Earthquake is a geological disaster with wide affected areas, strong destructiveness, and a large number of casualties, often causing enormous losses to humans and society in an instant.

Causes of casualties during earthquake include building collapse, gas leak, electric shock, drowning, and fire, among which building collapse is the most common.

On the premise of ensuring the safety of the rescue personnel, the principle of first near and then far, first rescue and then treatment should be followed at the scene, and carry out the integrated rescue of search, escape, rescue and medical treatment for people in the earthquake area.

Key Points of On-Site Rescue

(1) For survivors buried in the rubble, establish ventilation holes to prevent suffocation; after digging them out, immediately remove the foreign bodies from their mouths, noses, and bodies, and protect their eyes from light. Examine the survivors to determine their consciousnesses, respirations and circulations.

(2) When slowly rescuing the victims from the gap, keep their spine in a neutral position to avoid injury to the spinal cord.

(3) After rescuing the victims, immediately assess their injuries; prioritize those with acute and critical conditions such as loss of consciousness or severe bleeding, bandage wounds, stop bleeding, and fix fractures. Victims with spinal fractures should be transported correctly.

(4) Be especially attentive to victims with pre-existing heart disease or hypertension, as their condition may worsen or recur due to fear, potentially leading to sudden death.

(5) Self-rescue methods in dangerous environments

1) Avoid unstable collapsing objects or hanging objects above, use bricks, wooden sticks, or other materials to prop up walls to prevent being buried again during aftershocks.

2) Move nearby debris to expand your space.

3) Do not casually use indoor facilities, including power sources, water sources, do not use open flames.

4) Do not shout, conserve energy and call for help by tapping.

5) When you smell gas and odor, cover your mouth and nose with wet clothes.

6) Protect and save drinking water and food.

Earthquake Safety in Various Locations

General principles: Seek nearby shelter that can form triangular spaces; escape from dangerous places; avoid disaster-prone areas; cut off dangerous sources; avoid man-made accidents.

1. Indoor Earthquake Safety

Quickly take shelter near sturdy furniture or in areas where triangular spaces can be formed, such as inner wall feet and corners. If you are close to small spaces such as kitchens, bathrooms, or storage rooms, you can quickly hide inside. Do not jump out of windows, stand near windows, or go onto balconies.

2. School Earthquake Safety

(1) If outdoors, crouch down on the spot, protect your head with both hands, and avoid tall buildings or hazardous objects. Do not return to the classroom.

(2) If indoors, when the teacher signals to take cover, immediately protect your head and eyes with hands, and quickly hide under the desk. Do not jump out of windows or stand near windows or balconies during escape.

(3) Evacuate in an organized manner after the earthquake to avoid overcrowding.

3. Earthquake Safety in Public Places

Follow the instructions of on-site staff and crouch down beside sturdy objects nearby. Evacuate in an orderly manner, avoiding panic and overcrowding. Do not take elevators or stay in stairwells. In stadiums and theaters, crouch down or lie down beside the seats, avoiding hanging objects, and use backpacks or other items to protect your head. In shopping malls, bookstores, exhibition halls, and subway stations, crouch down beside sturdy counters, low furniture, columns, or inner wall corners, and use your hands or other items to protect your head. In the moving tram or car, clench handrails, lower your center of gravity, and take shelter near seats.

4. Outdoor Earthquake Safety

Crouch or lie down on the ground in an open area to avoid falling down, do not run around, and avoid crowded places; do not arbitrarily return indoors. Stay away from tall buildings, especially those with glass curtain walls; avoid pedestrian bridges, overpasses, tall chimneys, water towers, etc. Stay away from dangerous objects such as transformers, utility poles, streetlights, and billboards; avoid other hazardous areas such as narrow streets, dilapidated houses, dangerous walls, parapets, high gateways, areas under awnings, and places where bricks, tiles, and wood materials are piled up; avoid roads and railways.

Section 2   Fire

Overview

Fire refers to the disaster caused by the uncontrolled burning in time or space, which can cause certain damage to personal safety and property.

Key Points of On-Site Rescue

1. Do Not Enter Dangerous Areas or Be Greedy for Possessions

Life is the most important. Do not waste precious escape time in dressing or searching for and taking valuables because of shyness or concern for valuable items.

2. Simple Protection Is Essential

Homes and companies should be equipped with smoke masks. You can also cover your nose with a towel or a mask, wet your body with water, and crawl forward. Since smoke is lighter than air and floats in the upper part, escaping close to the ground is the best way to avoid inhaling smoke.

3. Slow Descent to Escape, Self-Rescue with a Rope

Do not blindly jump off buildings. Utilize the evacuation stairs, balconies, downpipes, etc., for self-rescue. You can also use ropes, bed sheets, curtains and clothes to make a simple life rope, wet it with water, tie it tightly to window frames, heating pipes, or railings, and protect your hands with towels or cloth strips to slide down or reach an unburned floor.

4. Act Decisively, Evacuate Quickly

When threatened by fire, put on wet clothes or bedding and escape towards a safety exit decisively. Do not blindly follow the crowd and avoid chaotic collisions. When evacuating, pay attention to escaping towards bright or open areas. Run downstairs when the fire is small; if the passage is blocked by smoke, turn your back to the smoke and escape to the rooftop or balcony.

5. Use the Passage Wisely, Avoid Elevators

Do not take elevators or escalators during a fire, but escape towards the safety exit.

6. Hold on and Wait for Help When a Big Fire Strikes

If the door feels hot, do not open it. If you open the door at this time, flames and smokes will come. Close doors and windows, use wet towels or cloth to block door gaps, or wet a quilt to cover doors and windows to prevent smoke infiltration and wait for rescuers.

7. Do Not Panic and Run if You Are on Fire

If you are on fire, do not run; instead, roll on the ground or use thick clothing to smother the flames.

8. Send Signals for Help

If all escape routes are blocked by fire, retreat indoors and use a flashlight, wave cloth, or call to send rescue signals to attract the attention of rescuers.

9. Familiarize Yourself with the Environment, Memorize Exits

Whether at home, school, shopping malls, or other public places, always pay attention to evacuation routes, safety exits, and stairway locations. When a fire starts and thick smoke is present, you can quickly find your way and escape the scene.

Section 3   Flood

Overview

Floods refer to disasters caused by extraordinary rainstorm or extreme high tides in coastal areas, causing rivers, oceans, and lakes to rise above a certain water level, resulting in damage to people, houses, farmland, factories, etc. in the flood-affected areas, threatening the safety of related areas and causing disasters to human society.

Key Points of On-Site Rescue

(1) When a flood arrives, first quickly climb to a sturdy high-rise building to avoid danger, then contact the rescue department, and pay attention to collecting floating materials such as wooden basins, barrels, and blocks as rescue equipment, which can be used to make wooden rafts in case of emergency.

(2) Shelters should generally be chosen as close to home as possible, at higher elevations, and with convenient transportation. Ideally, there should be water

facilities and good sanitary conditions. In cities, these are usually flat rooftops of high-rise buildings, sturdy schools, hospitals, and parks with high terrain.

(3) If time permits, prepare in advance. Store clean drinking water in wooden basins and other containers; prepare medical supplies and fire-starting items; storage clothing, quilts and other warm items in high places; bury the waterproof and bundle up valuable items that are difficult to carry in the ground or put them in high places; sew cash and jewelry into clothing.

(4) Preserve all available communication facilities, and maintain good communication and transportation connections with the outside.

(5) If the flood waters continue to rise and the temporary shelter can't protect safety, it is necessary to make full use of the prepared escape equipment, or quickly find some floating materials to form a raft to escape.

(6) If surrounded by floodwaters, try to contact the local flood control department as soon as possible, report your location and danger, and actively seek rescue. Note: Do not attempt to swim to escape, do not climb electrified poles or towers, and do not climb onto the roof of mud-brick houses. When high-voltage lines or towers are tilted, or wires are broken and hanging, quickly move away from the area.

(7) If caught in floodwaters, try to hold onto fixed or floating objects and look for opportunities to escape.

(8) In mountain areas, continuous heavy rain can cause flash floods. Be cautious about crossing rivers to avoid being swept away by flash floods, and pay attention to the risks of landslides, rolling stones, and mudslides.

(9) After the flood, carry out various sanitation and epidemic prevention measures to prevent the spread of diseases.

Section 4   Lightning Stroke

Overview

The contact point of lightning stroke is usually the point where the electric current enters and exits from the human body, and therefore mostly at the head, neck, or shoulders. Injured individuals may present burnt skin, ruptured tympanic membrane or internal organs, ventricular fibrillation, cardiac arrest, or respiratory muscle paralysis. After being struck by lightning, if there are no signs of cardiac arrest, the prognosis is generally good. Therefore, when multiple people are struck by lightning, priority should be given to patients who seem to be dead, and perform CPR in real-time, so that the heart and brain can receive oxygen quickly. Proper first aid can save lives and minimize the damage.

Key Points of On-Site Rescue

1. Prevention Is the Key to Lightning Stroke

Modern technology has been able to predict the occurrence of thunderstorms, so taking some measures can prevent the harm caused by lightning stroke.

(1) Avoid walking outdoors or taking shelter under large trees during thunderstorms. Remove metal objects from your body and squat down to avoid lightning.

(2) Stay away from lights and power sources during thunderstorms, and avoid being close to poles and walls to prevent induced electricity.

(3) Close doors, windows, and household appliances, and turn off the main power switch.

(4) If you are outdoors and feel your hair standing up, skin tingling, or muscles trembling, you may be in danger of being struck by lightning. Immediately squat down and try to minimize the contact area with the ground. Do not lie on the ground, especially on wet surfaces. These measures can effectively prevent lightning injuries or minimize the damage.

2. Lightning Stroke Usually Causes Sudden Cardiac Arrest

Immediately assess the patient, and if no chest movement is observed within 5 to 10 seconds, start CPR and call the emergency number "120".

Section 5　Elevator Emergencies

Overview

Elevator malfunctions usually cause psychological panic for trapped individuals. In such situations, do not act rashly, as the elevator may actually be safe.

Key Points of On-Site Rescue

(1) Regardless of the number of floors, quickly press all the buttons for each floor. When the emergency power is activated, the elevator can immediately stop its descent.

(2) When the elevator is falling, press your entire back and head against the elevator wall, forming a straight line. Use the elevator wall to protect your spine.

(3) If there is handrail in the elevator, firmly grasp it to stabilize your position and prevent injuries due to loss of balance. If there is no handrail, use your hands to support your neck to avoid neck injuries.

(4) Keep your knees bent, as ligaments are the most elastic tissues in the human body. Bending your knees can help withstand the impact of the force.

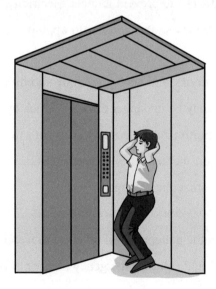

The best posture to protect yourself when the elevator falls

Avoid the following behaviors:

(1) Do not take excessive behavior, such as jumping in the elevator.

(2) Do not force the door open to climb out, in case the elevator starts suddenly.

Section 6　Outdoor Emergencies

Overview

Disasters or emergencies may happen unexpectedly in the wild, so it's necessary to master the skills of rescue in the wild. When in danger in the wild, you can use mobile phones and resources around you to send out distress signals. Making the distress target enlarged or distinctly different from the surrounding environment can more effectively convey the distress signal and help the victim rescued as soon as possible.

Outdoor Emergency Distress Signals

In case of distress in the wild, you can send out distress signals to the ground, sea, or air through the following methods, repeating three times to seek help.

1. Visual Signals

(1) Ground-to-air contact symbols. SOS is the internationally recognized emergency distress signal. You can also place HELP, SEND, DOCTOR, INJURY, TRAPPED, LOST, WATER, etc., in open spaces. Look for open grassland, snow, or beach to make ground marks, such as cutting grass into specific patterns or stomping out distress signals in the snow. You can also use branches, seaweeds, and other materials to create distress signals and make contact with the air.

(2) High-power flashlight. A high-power flashlight has three modes: strong light, weak light, strobe. The strobe mode is typically used for rescue.

(3) Pyrotechnic signal. The internationally recognized pyrotechnic distress signal is three fires arranged in an equilateral triangle. During the day, smoke is a good locator. Adding green grass, leaves, mosses, and ferns to the fire will produce

thick smoke. Wet straw mats or cushions can be used to produce smoke for a longer time. Black smoke is most noticeable in snow or deserts, rubber and gasoline can produce black smoke.

(4) Reflective signal. Using sunlight and a reflective mirror (such as glass or metal piece) can emit signal light. Continuous reflection will produce a long line and a dot regularly, which is a type of Morse code. Even if you don't understand Morse code, random reflection can also attract attention.

(5) Body indication signal. Stand on a high place and wave a piece of clothing with a contrasting color against the surrounding environment to express distress.

(6) Flag signal. Tie a flag or a piece of brightly colored cloth to a stick and move the stick: long stroke on the left side, short stroke on the right side, making an "8" shape movement.

2. Auditory Signals

Shout loudly or use a wooden stick to hit tree trunks or pipes. A rescue whistle is more effective, and the sharp whistle can attract the attention of rescuers. Remember that the whistle must have a rhythm, that is, three short, three long, three short, and repeat after a 1 minute interval.

3. Direction Indication Marks

Leave indication marks along the way to help rescuers find your path.

(1) Arrange rocks or broken stones into an arrow shape.

(2) Place sticks between the tree branches, with the top pointing in the direction of travel.

(3) Tie the knot in the middle and upper part of the grass, bending the top to indicate the direction of travel.

(4) Stack small stones into a large pile, with a small stone next to it pointing the direction of travel.

(5) Use an arrow-shaped groove that is carved into the tree trunk to indicate the direction of travel.

(6) Two crossed sticks or stones mean that the road is blocked.

(7) Use three rocks, sticks, or bushes to indicate danger or emergency signals.

Rescue Telephone Number

Police emergency: 110.

Fire emergency: 119.

Ambulance: 120.

Traffic accident emergency: 122; 12122 (Highway emergency).

Water rescue: 12395.

Urban construction service hotline (public transport, water supply, gas, heating, illegal construction, etc.) :12319.

Power supply service hotline: 95598.

Weather forecast hotline: 12121.

Red Cross emergency: 999.

Chapter 8

Psychological First Aid

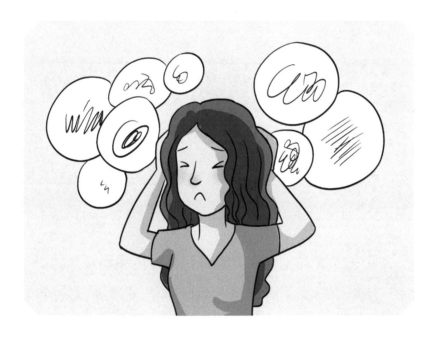

First aid should not only be focused on the body but also on psychology. If psychological trauma is not addressed, it may lead to insurmountable psychological barriers.

Psychological First Aid Kit

(1) "Medicines": fruits, tea, hometown food, green plants, flowers, perfume, music, etc.

(2) "Equipment": dolls, painting tools, calligraphy tools, swimming gear, badminton, hiking gear, etc.

(3) "Venues": indoors or outdoors.

(4) "Personnel": the person himself/herself, trusted teachers, friends, counselors, mental health professionals, psychological counselors, professional psychologists, etc.

Specific Steps for First Aid

(1) Cherish yourself: Remember that you are unique in the world, and life is precious. People may experience low emotional, frustration, failure, guilt, depression, rejection, separation, loss, anxiety, disappointment, inferiority, loneliness, social phobia, anger, helplessness, lost of love, unemployment, car accidents, and the passing away of loved ones. Everyone will encounter emotional trauma unexpectedly. Understand that all the pain we experience is understandable and reasonable.

(2) Master emotional trauma first aid skills: Emotional trauma, like physical trauma, requires self-treatment or hospital treatment. Seek treatment options to manage and soothe hurt emotions, invigorate your spirit, overcome setbacks, and break the cycle of negative energy.

(3) Choose to be strong: Believe that your emotional immune system can change bad emotions, suggest that you are a lucky person, regularly engage in emotional health care, maintain mental health, and have confidence in overcoming

difficulties and getting out of trouble.

(4) Set aside problems: You can refresh yourself by taking a bath and sleeping.

(5) Find and cultivate hobbies: Such as painting, calligraphy, photography, seal cutting, assembling toys, etc., or going out to watch movies, listen to cross talk, exercise, appreciate plants, flowers, music, etc., or raise pets, cultivate crops, or bonsai plants.

(6) Recuperate at home: Return to your hometown from a solitary residence, visit your parents, and work together to tidy up the home environment. Take care of elderly family members and nurture children. Cook food, bake, talk to relatives and friends, or quietly accompany them.

(7) Travel: Traveling allows you to experience and appreciate nature, enjoy beautiful scenery, or meet new friends.

Chapter 9

Pregnancy Health

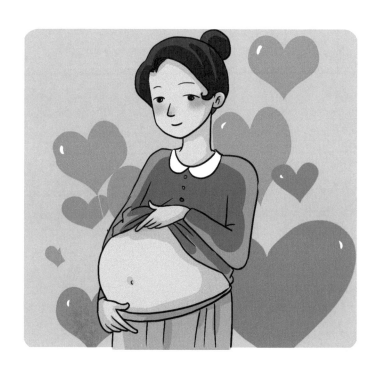

Overview

Prenatal health care involves active prevention, screening, monitoring, and health care throughout pregnancy to reduce and control the occurrence of certain diseases and genetic disorders, reduce maternal mortality rate, and promote women's physical and mental health.

Confirming Pregnancy

Cessation of menstruation is an important sign of pregnancy, but it does not necessarily indicate pregnancy. Pregnancy can only be confirmed after the examination at a regular hospital.

Expected Date of Confinement and Gestational Period

1. Expected Date of Confinement

Determine the date of the last menstrual period and estimate the expected date of confinement. Calculation method: from the first day of the last menstrual period, subtract 3 or add 9 months, and add 7 days; if using the lunar calendar, still subtract 3 or add 9 months, but add 15 days. The actual delivery date may differ from the expected date of confinement by 1 to 2 weeks.

2. Gestational Period

Gestational period is approximately 280 days (40 weeks) from the first day of the last menstrual period. Clinically, it is divided into three stages: early pregnancy from the beginning to 12 weeks, second trimester of pregnancy from 13 to 27 weeks, and late pregnancy from 28 weeks onward.

Common Pregnancy Symptoms

1. Early Pregnancy Symptoms

Early pregnancy symptoms include nausea, vomiting, frequent urination, increased vaginal discharge, etc. If vaginal bleeding occurs, seek medical attention promptly.

2. Second trimester and Late Pregnancy Symptoms

Second trimester and late pregnancy symptoms include edema, varices in the lower limbs and vulva, constipation, hemorrhoids, low back pain, lower limbs spasm, supine hypotension, insomnia, anemia, etc.

Prenatal Life Guidance

1. First and Last Three Months of Pregnancy

Avoid sexual activity to prevent abortion, premature birth, and infection.

2. Self-Monitoring During Pregnancy

1) Fetal heart sounds and fetal movement counting are important means for pregnant women to monitor the intrauterine condition of the fetus. Guiding pregnant women or family members to listen to fetal heart sounds correctly and keep records is not only helpful to understand the intrauterine development of the fetus, but also can promote affectionate relationships between family members.

2) Generally, pregnant women begin to feel fetal movement around 20 weeks of pregnancy. Fetal movement is usually more active at night and in the afternoon. Pregnant women can count fetal movements for 1 hour each in the morning, afternoon, and evening. There should be at least 3 fetal movements per hour, and a total of no less than 10 times within 12 hours.

3. Use of Medications

Many medications can pass through the placenta and affect embryo development, especially during the first 2 months of pregnancy. This is the period of embryonic organ development and formation, and pregnant women should be cautious when taking medications.

Principles of rational medication use for pregnant women:

Avoid combination of medications when one is sufficient; choose medications with proven efficacy, avoid those with uncertain adverse effects on the fetus; use small doses when possible, avoid large doses; strictly control dosage and duration, and discontinue medication timely. If necessary, terminate the pregnancy before using teratogenic medications harmful to the embryo and fetus.

4. Other Considerations

For example, when riding in a car, avoid having the seatbelt directly press against the abdomen, fasten it at the thigh root (groin).

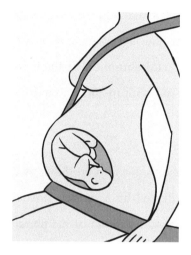

Correct seat belt position

Situations Requiring Immediate Medical Attention During Pregnancy

Pregnant women should seek immediate medical attention if they experience any of the following symptoms: severe vomiting or persistent vomiting after 3 months of pregnancy, headache, dizziness, chest distress, palpitations, shortness of breath, significant pitting edema in the lower limbs or can not relieve after rest, shivering and fever, abdominal pain, abnormal fetal movement, vaginal bleeding, premature rupture of fetal membranes, vaginal discharge, or a sudden decrease in fetal movement counts.

1. Abnormal Fetal Movement

After 28 weeks of pregnancy, if the fetal movements within 12 hours are less than 10 times or decreases more than 50% per day and does not recover, it suggests the possibility of fetal hypoxia in the uterus, and pregnant women should seek medical attention in time for further diagnosis and treatment.

2. Vaginal Bleeding

In early pregnancy, bright red vaginal bleeding with or without pain, may be related to threatened abortion, cervical lesions, extrauterine pregnancy, or hydatidiform mole, and medical attention should be sought promptly.

In the second trimester and late pregnancy, vaginal bleeding may be caused by placenta praevia or placental abruption. If there is vaginal bleeding, pregnant women should be vigilant and seek medical attention promptly regardless of the amount of bleeding.

3. Premature Rupture of Membranes

The rupture of fetal membranes before labor is called premature rupture of membranes, which is manifested by a sudden flow of fluid from the vagina in pregnant women. Once premature rupture of membranes occurs, pregnant women should take the supine position and be sent to the hospital by family members to prevent cord prolapse and endangering the life of the fetus.

Recognizing the Signs of Threatened Labor

Before delivery, some symptoms may indicate impending labor, such as irregular contractions, a feeling of fetus descent, and the appearance of a small amount of bloody discharge from the vagina (commonly known as "bloody show"). This is called threatened labor. Multiparas should seek medical attention as soon as they experience irregular contractions to prevent precipitous labor.

Regular contractions (with intervals of 5 to 6 minutes, lasting 30 seconds or more) that gradually intensify, accompanied by progressive cervical canal effacement, dilatation of cervix, and descent of the fetal presentation, are considered in labor, and pregnant women should seek medical attention as soon as possible.

Prehospital Emergency Delivery

With the implementation of the three-child policy, the situation of emergency delivery outside the hospital may increase. If pregnant women cannot be transported to the hospital in time for delivery and need a delivery on the spot, the following steps can be taken.

1. Pregnant Women Confirm Signs of Delivery

If a pregnant woman suddenly feels an uncontrollable urge to push, has a sense of defecation, and the sense becomes stronger and stronger, and even begins to feel that the fetus is going to fall out, indicating that the delivery is imminent.

2. Seek Assistance Immediately

The pregnant woman and her family members should call the emergency number "120" and seek assistance from the relevant personnel on-site.

3. Deep Breathing

When contractions begin, instruct the pregnant woman to take a deep breath through her nose, and then slowly exhale through her mouth, guiding her not to hold her breath and push too early.

4. Adjust Measures to Local Conditions

Rescuers should assess the scene and quickly place the pregnant woman in a nearby, safe, and hidden place, temporarily setting up a "obstetric bed". If there is a bed, spread a clean bed sheet and place a nursing pad or a clean towel under the pregnant woman's buttocks; if there is no bed, lay several clean clothes and towels on a relatively clean ground.

5. Lie Flat

The rescuers should ask the pregnant woman to lie on her back with her knees bent, remove any clothing that may interfere with delivery, and cover her body with clothing or other covers. Monitor the fetal head at the vaginal orifice.

6. Clean and Disinfect

If time permits, clean the pregnant woman's perineum with a cleanser or soapy water, and the hands of the person assisting the delivery should also be cleaned and disinfected. Wear gloves if possible (find substitutes on-site).

7. If the Fetal Head Is Not Visible

If the fetal head is not visible at the vaginal orifice, instruct the pregnant woman to lie on her left side, adjust her breathing, and not to push.

8. If the Fetal Head Is Visible

If the fetal hair or part of the head is visible at the vaginal orifice and the head is rapidly delivered out, instruct the pregnant woman to open her legs, take deep breaths, do not push, and prepare for delivery.

9. Help Deliver the Fetal Head

During the delivery of the fetal head, let the pregnant woman take quick, deep breaths. The midwife should support the fetal head with her/his left hand to control the speed of delivery and support the perineum (above the anus) with a clean, soft pad (or substitute) held in her/his right hand, allowing the fetal head to slowly slide out of the vagina. After the fetal head is delivered, gently squeeze the fetus's lower jaw upward with the left hand, and squeeze the root of nose downward with the right hand to expel mucus and amniotic fluid from the fetus's oral and nasal cavities.

10. Deliver the Shoulders

When waiting for the next contraction, gently press down the fetus's neck to deliver the front shoulder, and support the fetus's neck with the left hand to deliver the back shoulder. Do not pull forcefully. This process still requires the right hand to support and protect the perineum to prevent severe perineal tears. After both shoulders are exposed, support the body of the newborn to deliver slowly, properly secure to prevent falling to the ground.

11. After the Newborn Is Delivered

Wipe the newborn's mouth and nose with a clean gauze to remove mucus or blood, and immediately dry his/her body. Usually, newborns will cry on their own within 1 minute of birth. If the newborn does not cry, rub the back or pat the feet to stimulate crying. Loud crying indicates a clear airway.

12. Pay Attention to Umbilical Cord Handling

After the newborn cries, tie the umbilical cord tightly with clean clamps or strings at 15 cm and 20 cm from the root of the newborn's umbilical cord. Do not cut the umbilical cord arbitrarily.

13. Skin Contact

After the umbilical cord is handled, place the newborn on the mother's abdomen, with his/her abdomen facing down and head to one side. Cover the newborn and the mother with a clean towel and clothing.

14. Wait for the Placenta to be Delivered

Usually, the placenta can be delivered naturally within 5 to 15 minutes after the birth of the newborn. Do not forcefully pull the placenta. If there is minor vaginal bleeding, the umbilical cord can be pulled gently to deliver the placenta.

15. Placenta Disposal

After the placenta is delivered, place it carefully with the umbilical cord attached to one side. Do not cut and discard it.

16. Massage the Uterus

Gently massage the upper part of the uterus around the navel to promote contraction and hardening of the uterus, which can help reduce bleeding.

17. Postpartum Care

Rest in bed and keep warm while waiting for medical personnel.

Notes: To avoid dangerous situations, it is best not to leave the pregnant woman alone at home when delivery is approaching. In addition, as the expected date of delivery approaches, be prepared with hospital admission procedures and supplies for delivery, check the hospital driving route, and familiarize yourself with the admission process.

Chapter 10

Infection Control and Precaution Measures

Overview

First aid providers should pay attention to personal safety protection while providing emergency care, and take correct and effective preventive and safety measures to avoid cross-infection with patients. In addition, it is necessary to correctly understand the transmission routes of diseases based on standard precautions and increase the proper personal protection. Infectious diseases can be transmitted through air, droplets, and contact. Pathogens can spread through blood, body fluids, secretions, excretions, and vomitus. It is crucial to master the knowledge of transmission routes and protection points of infectious diseases.

Basic Protective Knowledge

1. Definition of Standard Precautions

Standard precautions refer to the belief that patients' blood, body fluids, secretions (excluding sweat), and excretions are infectious, and self-protection is required when in contact, regardless of whether there is obvious blood contamination or contact with non-intact skin and mucous membranes. Protective measures must be taken when contacting the above substances.

2. Measures of Standard Precautions

(1) First aid providers should wear gloves, and if conditions allow, wear masks, goggles, and isolation gowns when they may be exposed to splattered blood or body fluids during the rescue of patients.

(2) Be careful when handling sharp objects, and do not recap them.

(3) If sharp objects are used during the rescue process, they should be properly disposed of after use to prevent needle-stick injuries.

(4) First aid providers should perform hand hygiene after administering treatment. If gloves are worn, remove them and then perform hand hygiene. Wearing gloves cannot replace hand-washing.

Hand Hygiene Knowledge

If there is no obvious contamination on the hands, use a quick-drying hand sanitizer for hand hygiene; if there is obvious contamination, wash hands with running water.

1. Steps to Disinfect Hands with Quick-Drying Hand Sanitizer

(1) Take an adequate amount ($\geqslant 3$ml) of quick-drying hand sanitizer in the palm.

(2) Apply to both hands, making sure to completely cover all skin.

(3) Rub hands according to the six-step hand-washing method, adding wrist rubbing for at least 20 seconds, rubbing until thoroughly dry.

2. Steps to Wash Hands with Running Water

(1) Wet hands thoroughly under running water.

(2) Apply hand sanitizer (or soap) to both hands, covering all skin completely.

(3) Rub hands according to the seven-step hand-washing method for at least 15 seconds.

(4) Rinse.

(5) Dry.

The entire washing process should take 40 to 60 seconds.

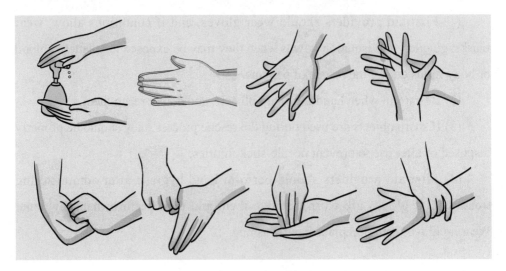

Hand hygiene guidelines

Protective Measures for Infectious Diseases with Different Transmission Routes

1. Air Transmission

Air transmission refers to the entire process of pathogens after being expelled from the source of infection and entering a new susceptible host through the air. Diseases transmitted through the air include tuberculosis, measles, and chickenpox. First aid providers must wear medical protective masks when treating such patients, remove the protective masks according to the specifications, and practice good hand hygiene.

Droplet transmission is a kind of air transmission, which refers to the way of disease transmission when the infected person releases pathogen-containing droplets from his/her mouth and nose when he/she is breathing, coughing, or sneezing, which are then inhaled by the susceptible person. It is the main transmission route for respiratory infections.

Diseases that can be transmitted through droplets include influenza, whooping cough, and severe acute respiratory syndrome (SARS). First aid providers should wear surgical masks, isolation gowns (if conditions allow), and practice good hand hygiene.

2. Contact Transmission

Contact transmission refers to the spread of pathogens through direct or indirect contact with a medium. Diseases that can be transmitted through contact include intestinal infections (diarrhea), multi-drug-resistant bacterial infections, and skin infections (impetigo). First aid providers should wear gloves, isolation gowns (if conditions allow), and practice good hand hygiene.

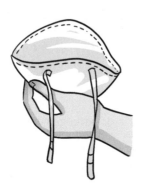
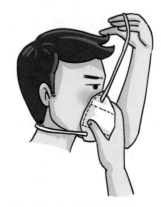

Wear medical protective mask correctly

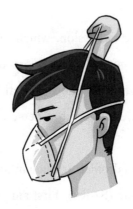
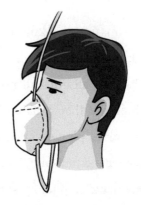

Remove medical protective mask correctly

Emergency Management After
Blood/Body Fluid Exposure

During first aid, emergency treatment is required for blood/body fluid exposure, different types of exposure require different treatment principles.

1. Needle-stick Injury

Rinse the wound under running water for about 5 minutes, then disinfect with iodophors or other disinfectants.

2. Skin and Mucosal Injury

Rinse the wound immediately and repeatedly with a large amount of running water or saline for at least 10 minutes.

All the above incidents should be reported to the hospital infection control department immediately for treatment.

Handling and Disposal of Contaminated Objects and Waste

After completing the rescue procedures, all first aid objects that can be discarded after use and wastes must be discarded in designated plastic bags, packed and sealed, and if conditions allow, handed over to professionals for classification and disposal according to the categories of domestic waste and medical waste.